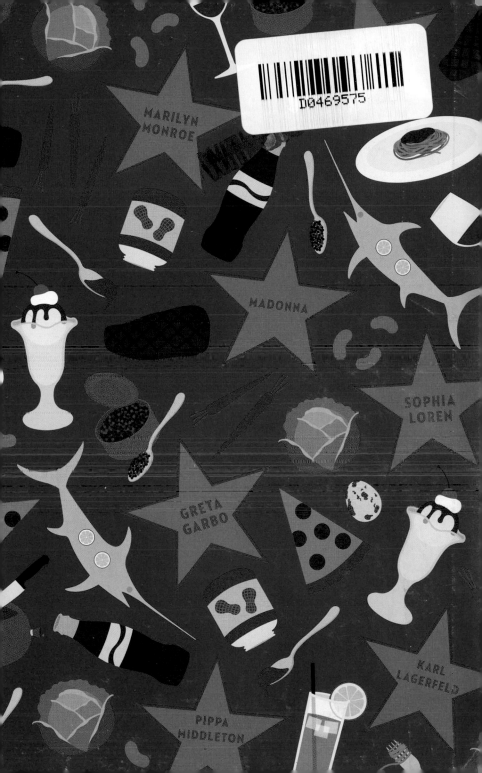

Rebecca Harrington

I'LL HAVE WHAT SHE'S HAVING

Rebecca Harrington is the author of the novel *Penelope*. She studied history and literature at Harvard and journalism at Columbia. Her work has appeared in *New York* magazine, the *New York Times*, and other publications and on NPR.com. She lives in New York City.

I'LL HAVE WHAT SHE'S HAVING

My Adventures in Celebrity Dieting

Rebecca Harrington

VINTAGE BOOKS

A Division of Random House LLC · New York

A VINTAGE ORIGINAL, JANUARY 2015

The following pieces originally appeared on the *New York* magazine blog "The Cut" (nymag.com/thecut): "Beyoncé's Diets Are the Most Effective I Have Ever Tried"; "Madonna's Diet Is the Hardest I Have Ever Tried"; "I Tried Gwyneth Paltrow's Diet"; "I Tried Greta Garbo's Strange, Horrifying Diet"; "I Ate Haggis and Aqua-Cycled on the Pippa Middleton Diet"; "Raw Eggs in Milk? Trying Marilyn Monroe's Diets"; "Cottage Cheese Mixed with Sour Cream? I Tried the Liz Taylor Diet"; "I Tried Jackie Kennedy's Caviar Diet"; and "I Tried Carmelo Anthony's Infamous Diet, and It Was Pathetically Easy."

Library of Congress Cataloging-in-Publication Data
Harrington, Rebecca.
I'll have what she's having: : my adventures in celebrity dieting / Rebecca Harrington. — First vintage edition.
pages cm
1. Weight loss.   2. Reducing diets.   3. Celebrities—Nutrition.
I. Title.
RM222.2.H249 2015   613.2'5—dc23   2014017817

**Vintage Trade Paperback ISBN: 978-1-1018-7243-7
eBook ISBN: 978-1-1018-7244-4**

Illustrations by Joan Wong
Book design by Jaclyn Whalen

www.vintagebooks.com

Printed in the United States of America
10 9 8 7 6 5 4 3 2 1

To my grandmother,
who always encouraged my love of old movies
and is constantly glamorous
without even eating a quail egg

Contents

A JOURNEY BEGINS   5

I Tried Gwyneth Paltrow's Diet   13

I Tried Elizabeth Taylor's Diet   27

I Tried Karl Lagerfeld's Diet   39

I Tried Marilyn Monroe's Diet   49

I Tried Cameron Diaz's Diet   59

I Tried Madonna's Diet   69

I Tried Greta Garbo's Diet   79

I Tried Victoria Beckham's Diet   91

I Tried Beyoncé's Diet   101

I Tried Jackie Kennedy's Diet   111

I Tried Sophia Loren's Diet   121

I Tried Pippa Middleton's Diet   131

I Tried Carmelo Anthony's Diet   143

I Tried Dolly Parton's Diet   151

AND NOW, A SLICE OF PIZZA   159

ACKNOWLEDGMENTS   163

I'LL HAVE WHAT SHE'S HAVING

Food is an important part of a balanced diet.

—FRAN LEBOWITZ

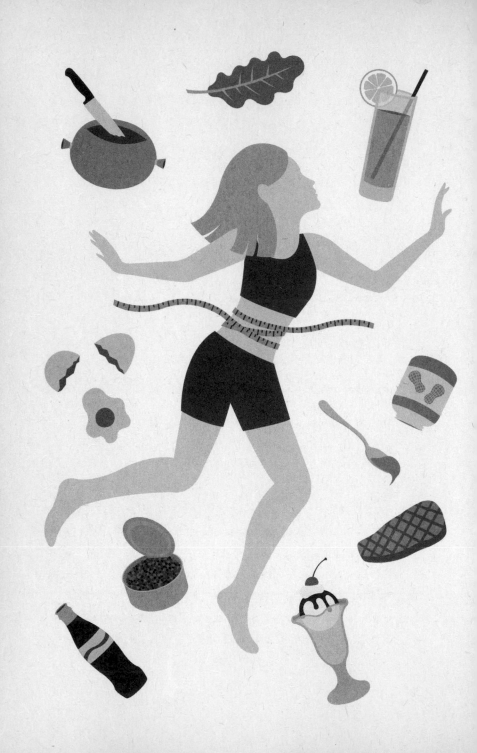

A Journey Begins

I have always noticed diets. Diets are everywhere. You can't be a woman and not think you need to go on a diet or get a face transplant. Preferably the face of a famous person so that you can never get lost. But noticing diets is completely different from doing many of them in succession. Who would do that? Me. Here is the story.

The first diet I ever went on was William Howard Taft's diet. William Howard Taft was America's fattest president, and I found his diet on this sleep apnea website that someone sent me. This sleep apnea website was convinced that "no president with the possible exception of Lincoln has faced greater challenges" than Taft because he might have had sleep apnea. Actually, they are still not sure whether he actually had sleep apnea or not. He was always falling asleep at the card table.

A small part of the website was devoted to a diet Taft went on in 1905. Taft had always been appointed to posts because people liked him (even though his best friend *and* his wife wrote books about how they hated him), and at this point he had just been appointed secretary of war by Roosevelt and wanted to be seen in fighting condition. So he went on a diet that called for boiled fish in the morning, mutton at night, and glutinous biscuits for snacks. He lost a bunch of weight because that is disgusting.

This diet obsessed me. Why? I don't know. I went on it for no reason. The hardest part was the glutinous biscuits. I had to make them from scratch, and I used a shampoo bottle to roll out the dough. Sometimes I would read the letters of Major Archibald Butt, Taft's best friend who hated him. But mostly I boiled sole for breakfast and ate it with Worcestershire sauce.

After I enjoyed boiled fish in the morning for a decent amount of time, I started to tell my friends about the new cool diet I was on that was making me lose no weight.

Some seemed confused about why I would be so interested in the eating habits of Taft. ("It's because he had
a cow named Pauline!" I would say.) Others suggested I
do regular diets of real celebrities that people were interested in, and since I had decided that celebrity eating
seemed a lot odder than normal eating, I agreed, and my
diet adventure was born.

What is the enduring fascination with celebrity eating?
One of the strangest things about researching these diets
was how easy it was to find out what famous people eat
every day. People are obsessed! It is practically the only
thing you can find when researching actresses. That and
how fun it is to work with someone who seems vaguely
boring.

Not content to leave such business to *Us Weekly*, many
modern celebrities have chosen to monetize their eating
habits themselves, releasing cookbooks and workouts and
various other lifestyle trinkets. Their nutritional regimens
are now part of the business of being a celebrity. In our
current antigluten, GMO-phobic culture, this often means
celebrities must espouse a "healthy," "non-processed" lifestyle, even if they are lying and actually keep their bodies
in shape with a combination of excellent genes and ciga-

rettes. I suppose celebrities are providing a road map for imitating them. And when telling us how to imitate them, sharing an eating plan is so much easier than offering up a screed about genes and cigarettes—not to mention more attainable, less jealousy-inducing, and more marketable. If you knew that eating goji berries would make you look like Jessica Biel, why wouldn't you do it?

I became interested in the diets of celebrities not necessarily because I wanted to have the ideal body (I already knew I was too squat, like a partridge waddling across a field) but because I really do like movies and I have always enjoyed doing experiments on myself in the style of Benjamin Franklin. I suppose it is the Enlightenment philosopher within me. Although, my experiences with the diets were probably closest to *Confessions of an English Opium-Eater* rather than any other seminal text of literature. I ate and then I discussed the aftereffects of what I ate with a barely suppressed glee and a pretend hatred.

Here are the rules I set for myself: I would try to eat the way celebrities normally eat. While it could be amusing to try to imitate the life-threatening efforts made by Christian Bale to slim down to the size of a Popsicle stick for *The Machinist*, it wasn't scientific enough for me, Ben Franklin. I would also buy any cookbook a celebrity wrote, even if it looked really bad. And I would try to employ exercise regimens, clothing choices, or dinner parties when appropriate.

But when faced with the almost Herculean task of dieting like a celebrity for an extended period of time and reporting on it, I had to ask myself a certain number of questions. What would happen to me after going on a million celebrity diets? Would I live? Would my friends stay with me until the end even though I kept making them come to my house for dinner parties where they all told me to my face that they despised all of my food? Would I get a rash on my cheek and would it clear up? Could I achieve my ideal body? My ideal personality (a combo of Liz Taylor and Liz Taylor)? I also wanted to answer what always seemed to be either a genius rhetorical question or a question that made absolutely no sense: Are you what you eat?

Actually, the idea that you are what you eat may have come from Ludwig Feuerbach—a respectable philosopher George Eliot translated into English. Or it may have come from a great eater and dieter, Jean Anthelme

Brillat-Savarin, who was both the founder of the low-carbohydrate diet and the writer of several tomes about gastronomy. Is the idea a philosophical meditation on the process of imbibing or the siren call of the celebrity dieter? I was about to find out!

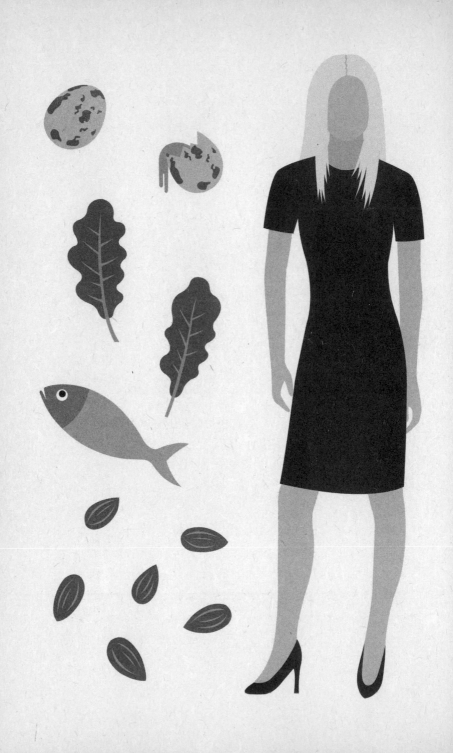

I Tried
Gwyneth Paltrow's Diet

I have always been an admirer of Gwyneth Paltrow—I am not afraid to admit it. She was so good in my favorite movie, *A Perfect Murder*. I also think her secondary career as a lifestyle guru is rather inspiring. If there wasn't a *Goop*, I would not have an eye mask that has hollow indentations so that you can blink.

When Gwyneth came out with her newest cookbook, *It's All Good*, I was very excited. I had her other cookbook, *My Father's Daughter*, already. It's a really good cookbook for the average woman (me). There are some healthy recipes and there are some delicious recipes. One time I had a dinner party and I made beer-battered fish tacos from that book and everyone liked them. This is saying a lot because usually my dinner parties are miserable failures in which people start ordering sushi in front of me like I'm not even there.

This new cookbook of Gwyneth's has an interesting genesis. After enduring a panic attack during a supper party (I really understand), Gwyneth went to several doctors and realized she had sensitivities to various foods, such as dairy, gluten, and chickens' eggs. Thus, she felt she had to make a cookbook that eliminated all the bad foods that ruin lives, like bread, deep-water fish, red meat, cow's milk, and eggplant, and focus on the "good" foods in the world, like goji berries and quail eggs. Hence *It's All Good*! Do you get it? All the foods that are not bad.

I was eager to try this diet for many reasons. I always think I have allergies to mysterious foods. Plus this is a diet written by a woman who almost convinced me to buy really expensive towels from the country of Turkey because they were more absorbent. I basically signed up fifteen years ago when I watched *A Perfect Murder* for the first time.

Preparation

I go online and purchase Gwyneth's book as well as Tracy Anderson's Method DVDs. Gwyneth reportedly does Tracy Anderson's fitness routine, which focuses on "small muscles," for two hours a day, so if I am going to live Gwyneth, I figure I might as well try to get her butt—that of a twenty-two-year-old stripper. When I finally get the book a month later (I preordered it like a weirdo), I am filled with both happiness and fear. The book itself is beautiful; there are all these pictures of Gwyneth in a floppy hat in front of a barn or Gwyneth putting a huge fish in a vat of salt. While doing a close reading, however, I am stunned at the magnitude of the things I will have to give up. I can't even eat yogurt! Nor can I have a tomato or a strawberry! They all cause allergies! It seems excessive to me, yet the book also promises me that if I do this, I will have Gwyneth's "clear eyes, glowing skin and fit body." And I definitely want clear eyes! I decide to follow the seven-day detox diet listed in the back of the book, as well as a smattering of her other diet menus. One day I will live like a vegan Gwyneth; another day I will eat like a child of Gwyneth. Hopefully this will give me the whole Gwyneth experience.

Next, I go food shopping. I have been on many diets before, but I have never paid this much for a week of groceries in my entire life. At $154.31, it is almost triple what I usually pay for food, and I haven't even bought all the fish I will eventually need! (The diet is really heavy on fish.) I bought at least ten dollars' worth of kale and an eleven-dollar jar of honey. Do you know what raw honey is? It is eleven dollars! I actually had a mild panic attack while buying the food and I wasn't even having a dinner party.

Day 1

Every day on the Gwyneth diet starts with a heaping helping of something called "The Best Green Juice." Like lots of other green juices, it is a mixture of kale, apple, lemon, mint, and ginger. I imagine it would be much easier to make this juice if you have a juicer, but I don't have one of those. Gwyneth says it is equally fine to make with a blender and a "fine mesh strainer," which I also don't think I have. Since I literally cannot spend any more money for a year, I will have to do without. I put the ingredients in the blender and blend them together. It tastes much like regular kale juice except it has large pieces of kale still in it. This is breakfast.

After breakfast, I decide to do the first DVD of the Tracy Anderson Method. It's difficult, actually. Essentially you hold tiny weights in your hands and then flap your arms wildly like a person in a Victorian insane asylum having an epileptic fit. You do this for an hour. At the end, I am so tired I lie on the floor.

After my workout, I decide to eat my morning snack—raw almonds soaked in water. Wet almonds are better than dry almonds because, according to Gwen, regular almonds are "hard to digest." Wet almonds sound gross but are actually delicious. The almonds have a kind of vanilla flavor to them once you soak them. I never really liked almonds before this. Is this diet actually going to be okay?

After a hearty lunch of a beet-greens soup (a soup made of the green leaves attached to a beet?) and an afternoon smoothie that combines both avocado and cocoa powder (this is sort of like ice cream if ice cream tasted like avocados), I invite my friend over for Gwyneth's version of barbecued chicken. My friend is usually quite skeptical of my diet experiments but is an incredibly good sport. I once made her eat a bean stew I made, for example, and we are still friends today. This time, however, I shock her. "This is really good!" she says, almost taken aback. It is true. It's really good chicken. It's juicy and has an interesting flavor from the paprika Gwyneth had me use. I have eaten so healthily the entire day, it was all super delicious, and I was not even hungry. I'm starting to feel slightly superior. "You should soak raw almonds in water," I say to my friend.

Day 2

Flush with last night's success, I decide to hold a dinner party at my home and fix on making Gwyneth's meatballs, which do not have bread, eggs, red meat, or milk in them. My mother makes very good meatballs, and those four things are basically the only ingredients in them, so I find this recipe suspect, but I press on. I thought wet almonds would be terrible, but I was wrong about that. I don't know how to live!

While making the meatballs, however, I can tell something is up. Number one: They are green (they are made of arugula and turkey). Number two: I can't put them in tomato sauce because I have eliminated tomatoes from my diet. Instead, I am serving them with a broccoli soup that tastes mostly like water. What is going on? Yesterday was so amazing! When my guests arrive and I feed them the meatballs,

I can tell that they hate them. One of them pulls out a huge bag of chips and starts eating them in front of me. Another one leaves to "actually eat dinner." I am about to have a panic attack when I remember when Gwyneth went to a dinner party in America and someone asked her what kind of jeans she was wearing and she thought to herself, "I have to get back to Europe." America is the worst. I say nothing about anyone's jeans, even though I was literally just going to ask everyone about their jeans.

Days 3 and 4

This diet is much harder on the weekends. This city is stupid because everyone is obsessed with gluten-filled brunch and what even is it? Just an empty parade! I have to get back to Europe. On Sunday, I get to go to a pancake place that also sells kale juice, and I silently watch my friend eat a pancake as I sip on some kale juice. Later, however, I roast a whole fish and serve it with anchovy salsa verde. It's absolutely delicious. "I would like to meet Gwyneth Paltrow," says a friend eating the fish with a large spoonful of anchovy sauce. "She sounds really fun." I enthuse: "She's so fun. She smokes one cigarette a week!"

Day 5

Deep in the bowels of my kitchen, I find something amazing. It is called a fine mesh strainer! I must have bought it when I was in a coma. Now my kale juice tastes just like kale juice. The homemade horchata I make for a midmorning snack is deeply improved. You really need raw honey for it, actually. It tastes much better and is non-alkaline forming. What has become of me?

Days 6 and 7

On the days when you are not waving your arms like a loon, Tracy Anderson has another DVD called *Dance Cardio Workout*. It's so incredibly hard that I can only do twenty minutes of it. From what I can gather, it is completely unexplained jumping to the dulcet beeping of late Madonna. You have to jump for a whole hour. I'm so tired afterward I actually have to go to sleep.

For dinner the next night, I make salt-roasted fish. You take a fish, cover it with herbs, and literally pour an entire container of salt on it. It's okay. I think the whole thing would have been better if I really loved Thai chilies, but I don't really like them that much. Sometimes, when I am cooking these recipes, I talk to my Gwyneth book like it is her incarnate. For example, I will say, "That's a lot of salt, Gwyneth," or "Goji berries *are* better when they are soaked in water. Thanks, buddy!"

This is the last day of my detox, and I have to say, it was kind of the best! I was never hungry, I loved almost all of the food I cooked, and I am actually much less swollen under my eyes than usual. I even feel slightly more alert, probably because I am not eating any tomatoes.

Day 8

Today, I try out Gwyneth's vegan food. Her vegan sesame pancakes are a delight. They taste like regular sesame pancakes except they have no gluten or dairy. Gwyneth's version of veganism is not very different from her detox diet. It just has absolutely no meat or animal stuff. Did you know that Gwyneth had a vegan-themed party for her daughter Apple's birthday? The more you know.

Day 9

One time Gwyneth told the New York *Daily News* that she would "rather die than let [her] kid eat Cup-a-Soup." This leads me to ask the question: Would it be fun to eat like a child of Gwyneth? Guess what? It's really fun! For breakfast, I make her "buttermilk" (they are vegan and gluten-free and have lemon juice and soy milk instead of buttermilk) pancakes. They are actually quite delicious, if slightly gummy. Her tuna salad with Vegenaise and Dijon mustard is decent and respectable! It is good, so far, to be Apple and Moses, and not just because they pick avocados all the time and eat wood-grilled pizza.

For dinner, I decide to redeem myself and hold a dinner party again, this time making tacos the main event. Who doesn't like tacos? I also decide to make an eggless and dairyless cake. The tacos are a stunning success. Gwyneth's recipe for homemade chipotle salsa is as good as what I would eat at the actual Chipotle. I am very proud of her and I cannot hide it. When people compliment the tacos, I say things like, "It's Gwyneth!" or "This cookbook is really great. I don't know how she does it." I don't ask one person about their jeans. The cake, however, is another matter. It's crumbly and tastes like a prune, but this is probably my fault. "I like the tacos," one of my friends says, after I ask about the cake.

Day 10

I have consciously uncoupled from the Gwyneth diet and lost four pounds in the process. I have much more defined arms from having hysterical fits every day. It is definitely fun to eat bread, dairy, and eggs again, but when I finally have all those things for the first time after ten days without them, I wake up with a huge rash down the side of my face, like the Phantom of the Opera. Have I always actually been allergic to these foods? The rash goes away eventually, but I do feel suddenly distrustful of bread.

What have I learned from Gwyneth's diet? It's an awesome way to live! If I wasn't going to go bankrupt doing it, I would follow the Gwyneth diet to the letter every day. The food is healthy, delicious, and filling; the recipes are not particularly complicated; and you avoid a huge rash on your face that you apparently just lived with before. If this is the way the other half lives, I want to live it! Let's all appreciate that she shares her awesome tips with the world.

One time, Gwyneth went to Arizona for a spiritual retreat. She was walking in the Sedona mountains, and the rocks told her, "You have the answers. You are your teacher." I agree with those rocks.

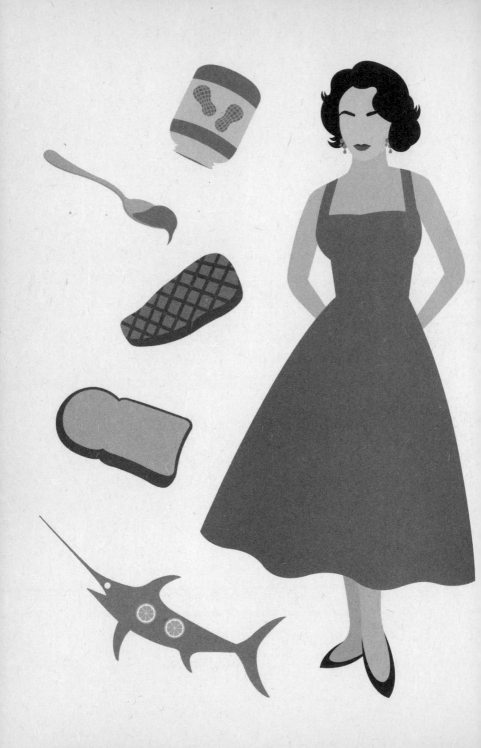

I Tried
Elizabeth Taylor's Diet

In 1960, when she was generally considered to be the most beautiful woman in the world, Elizabeth Taylor's daily diet consisted of the following: Scrambled eggs, bacon, and a mimosa for breakfast. A hollowed-out piece of French bread filled with peanut butter and bacon for lunch. And for dinner, a feast: fried chicken, peas, biscuits, gravy, mashed potatoes, corn bread, homemade potato chips, trifle, and a tumbler full of Jack Daniel's.

But like all great eras in history, the age of Taylor's high-calorie eating habits came to an end. During her fifth marriage, she gained quite a bit of weight, eventually reaching "180-odd pounds," and then lost it, plummeting to 121 pounds (she reached 119, realized she was losing her bust, and "put on some flesh in a hurry!"). In 1987, she wrote a diet book called *Elizabeth Takes Off.* The cover of the book has a picture of Liz staring off into space as if transfixed by a magnet. It was a national bestseller and is now out of print.

As a die-hard fan of both diets and Liz Taylor, I was curious to test her eating plan. How could a woman who appreciated the best of everything—food, furs, men, diamonds—create a bad diet? She couldn't. Or so I thought.

Preparation

In the days leading up to the diet, I start to read *Elizabeth Takes Off.* "It's too easy to become fixated on calories," Liz writes breezily. I nod. "Too tempting to say to yourself, 'Umm . . . I can have 20 potato chips for 230 calories, or 6 oz. of chicken for 310 calories' . . . That's no way to lose weight." This sounds correct to me. Math has always been a personal scourge. As I flip through the recipes, though, I become worried. Cottage cheese with sour cream? Steak with peanut butter on it? Dry toast every single morning? This sounds very disgusting, but who am I to question Liz? She says she is "rarely hungry" on her diet.

The book itself is not particularly concerned with food, really, despite the fact that it is ostensibly a book about dieting. There are a lot of pictures and chapters about Liz's personal life. She thinks she married so many times because of her "quaint attitudes." "Basically I'm square," she says. Me too, Elizabeth!

Day 1

Every breakfast on the Liz Taylor diet is the same: dry toast and a piece of fruit. Dry toast is a weird thing, I must say. Like a cracker with a strangely moist interior. This morning, I can't deal with the toast, so I eat only the fruit. In an hour I am ravenous. For dinner, I prepare a fillet of swordfish using Liz's recipe, which is essentially to sprinkle lime juice on the swordfish and stick it in the oven. It tastes like a lime-flavored old shoe on the ground.

The one bright spot is that I am not compelled to exercise. Liz's feelings on physical fitness are ambivalent at best; one chapter of this book is titled "Aerobic Exercises: Are They for You?" One exercise is to stand on your toes.

Day 2

For dinner this evening, I am supposed to make a piece of steak and put it on top of a piece of bread slathered with peanut butter. Despite being so hungry I could eat my hand, I cannot handle this concoction. The steak's juices mix with the peanut butter in an unappealing, oily way. I have three bites, then throw the rest out.

Elizabeth Takes Off advocates several mental dieting techniques, such as pinning a picture of yourself at your fattest on your fridge. Apparently Liz heard that Debbie Reynolds used a fat picture of her this way, after Liz stole Debbie's husband. (Eddie Fisher was Debbie's first husband and Liz's fourth.) "If you think this picture of me as Miss Lard will inspire you," Liz writes, "go ahead and put it on your refrigerator, I have no objection." I refrain from tearing Liz's picture out of my book but spend some time clicking through photos of myself on Facebook. They are all unflattering.

Day 3

On the third day of the diet, I become so hungry that I decide to make one of Liz Taylor's famous dips. You are supposed to have dip every day at 3:00 p.m. with a series of raw vegetables. And so, in the afternoon, I mash sour cream, blue cheese, vinegar, and a shallot together. I dip a piece of broccoli into it and eat it. It's not bad, but it does make me rather conspicuous in my office. The dip smells vaguely of rotting eggs, and later I introduce myself to someone, casually holding a piece of broccoli with dip on it the entire time. I think about this a lot throughout the day. "Why didn't I just put down the broccoli?" I ask myself, and cannot come up with any sort of answer. Suffice it to say, it does not remind me of the time when Mike Todd (Liz's third husband) said to her, "Why, honey, you're a latent intellectual," when they first met on a yacht.

That evening I host a dinner party. I make tacos for my guests and Liz's ratatouille for myself. The recipe consists of vegetables boiled to a goop in tomato paste and eaten with a spoon. It is nothing like the French food in that Pixar movie. (Was anyone else grossed out that rats made the ratatouille? Even though that is a pun, I still hate it.)

Bright spot: I do make Liz's favorite cocktail, which she used to drink with Rock Hudson on the set of *Giant*. Apparently filming *Giant* was just the worst, and in an effort to "bolster [their] spirits," Rock and Liz drank all the time. It was during one of these "toots" (?) that Liz made what she termed "the best drink [she] ever tasted"—a combination of Hershey's syrup, vodka, and Kahlúa. Everyone at my party hates the drink, but I like it because it's the most logical flavor combination I've had in days.

Day 4

I have now realized I *love* dry bread. It's so delicious; why didn't I know this before? It is by far the best thing I have eaten.

Days 5, 6, and 7

Liz is a big believer in what she calls a "controlled pig-out." She says it really helped her stay on the wagon with her diet. A controlled pig-out is when you eat everything you want, indulging your "wildest food fantasies" for one meal a day. For example, on one of Liz's controlled pig-outs, she ate a whole pizza followed by a hot-fudge sundae.

For my controlled pig-out, I eat like the old Liz. I have a peanut butter and bacon sandwich and fried chicken.

They are delicious, but then I get incredibly sick after I have them. Perhaps my stomach shrank from lack of food.

Day 8

I'm supposed to eat fillet of sole for dinner, but I have a date with some friends. I force everyone to go to an abandoned restaurant, the only place in the vicinity that serves sole. I am loudly derided for this, and I don't actually blame my friends because I have flagrantly disobeyed one of Liz's cardinal rules. "When you are dieting, be discreet," she writes. "You don't have to report to your acquaintances as though they were the commanding officers of your Great War Against Fat. Even your most supportive friends can become bored."

I fear that my friends have become very bored with me after the sole incident. They all eat mozzarella sticks rather sourly while I talk about how sole is okay if you don't stuff it with crabmeat and yet how it pains me to take the crabmeat out of the sole because I am too hungry to deprive myself of any calories. I am so famished when I get home that I make "minted new potatoes," a swampy mess of mint leaves and potatoes.

Days 9, 10, and 11

I go on vacation to Cape Cod with my family. My mother says I look thin but is grossed out by the dip I am eating. Every night my family eats something delicious, like spaghetti and meatballs, and I eat something separate and disgusting, like overcooked swordfish. I go to the beach and stare into the ocean, thinking about food and how much I miss it. This must be the opposite of how Taylor Swift feels when she is in Cape Cod.

Days 12 and 13

Sheer hunger drives me to combine cottage cheese and sour cream and pour it over fruit, as Liz recommends. (Previously I left out the sour cream.) It resembles curdled milk and tastes similar. Absolutely repugnant. Never try it.

Stray observations: Plain veal is extremely disgusting, a bit like eating a cardbord box that has been left out in the sun. Nutmeg on vegetables is problematic. Liz's attitude is wearing off on me, though. I find myself imitating Liz's style, as documented in the photo section of her book. In tighter clothes and bigger earrings, I contemplate marrying a hotelier or Shakespearean actor. I don't know where to go to meet them, though. Maybe an airport.

Day 14

I decide to make Liz's tuna salad. This recipe combines tomato paste with tuna, grapefruit, scallions, and mayonnaise. Do these disparate flavors act like an experiment in molecular gastronomy? No, they do not. It is more similar to something a cat would like.

Day 15

I finish the diet! I jump on my mother's scale and find that I am six pounds lighter. I am also hungrier than I have ever been in my life.

I have also gained a new appreciation for Liz Taylor's irrepressible personality. Even as she describes the most disgusting meals imaginable in *Elizabeth Takes Off*, Liz is funny and self-deprecating, unapologetic about her marriages, and a total gossip about her extensive web of friends and her hatred of Louis B. Mayer.

She is, in short, an excellent broad with really bad taste in food.

At the end of one chapter, Liz describes a recent birthday party. As party favors, Liz gave each female guest a rhinestone reproduction of the Taylor-Burton diamond. "Camp, yes, but I loved it," Liz enthused. That is pretty much how I feel about her diet.

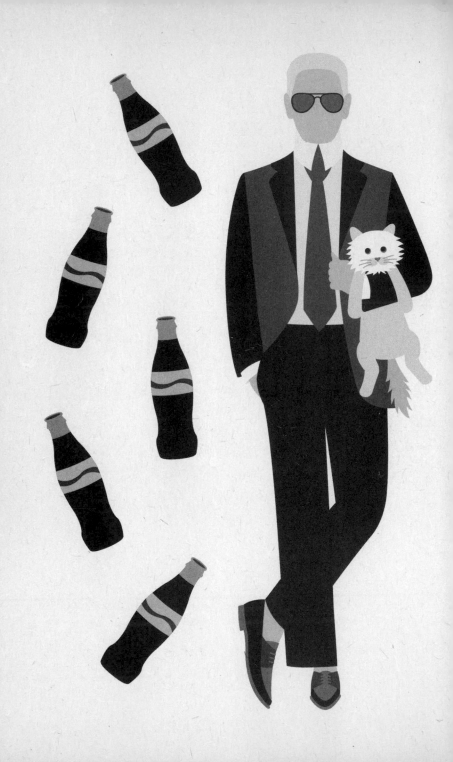

I Tried
Karl Lagerfeld's Diet

Most people think of Karl Lagerfeld, the head designer for Chanel, as a whippet-thin man with a shock of white hair. This wasn't always so. Though he has always had white hair (Karl loves the eighteenth century because everyone had white hair then), nineties Karl was far plumper and wore diaphanous jackets with a huge wooden fan around his neck. He looked rather jolly actually, or would have if the fan was not there.

With the new millennium on the horizon, however, Karl decided to lose a bunch of weight. He claims it was entirely for "superficial reasons." Apparently Karl was seized with the desire to "dress differently [and] to wear clothes designed by [Dior Homme's] Hedi Slimane."

However, he also realized that "these fashions . . . would require [him] to lose 80 pounds." After devoting himself to a strict diet designed by weight-loss guru Dr. Jean-Claude Houdret, he lost all the weight within the year. This dramatic weight loss was so remarked upon in the fashion community that Lagerfeld wrote a book about it, entitled *The Karl Lagerfeld Diet*. It was a bestseller in France because how could it not be?

Karl Lagerfeld has a cat named Choupette that I have always liked (she knows how to use an iPad and she has two lady's maids, one for day and one for night), so I wanted to attempt the Karl Lagerfeld diet as a way of congratulating her. Also, anything that involves losing eighty pounds in a year must be effective, at the very least.

Preparation

I purchase Karl's book and lug it home from the bookstore. The cover shows Karl in boot-cut jeans he would probably glower at now, looking fiercely at the corner of the book jacket. He seems both mad and ready to diet, as am I.

After a particularly long period of contemplating the book's cover, much the way a five-year-old Karl obsessively contemplated a painting of white-haired eighteenth-century aristocrats in his family's home, I open the book. Inside there is a large picture of Lagerfeld's diet doctor, Dr. Jean-Claude Houdret, who has a long Salvador Dalí–style mustache with curled ends. Dr. Houdret is the creator of the Spoonlight program—a French diet that advocates a mix of very expensive protein packets and meager bits of food. He actually wrote most of Karl's diet book, it turns out. The book is written in a very high-literary style for a diet book, I must say. The conclusion is a meandering essay on the way a dandy functions in modern society. One would think the good doctor would know something about that because of his mustache.

Which is not to say that Karl had no hand in writing the book that bears his name; he did. Karl's passages turn up occasionally, helpfully signed with his initials, KL. Karl is also interviewed at the beginning of the book by Ingrid Sischy, where he explains the genesis of his diet, and how he can't even remember the man he was two years ago when he was fat, and that he's so disciplined he's not even tempted by any foods. Aside from the interview (which is very long and slightly repetitive), there are several essays on cosmetic surgery and skin care and personal anecdotes of a young and inexperienced medical professional by Dr. Salvador Dalí. Eventually, I find a brief description of the actual diet tucked in the middle of the book. There are several different diets the doctor prescribes—including a nine-hundred-calorie one that consists entirely of protein "sachets" and vegetables for the very severe weight-loss cases. I decide to pass on this as I have put myself through enough in the years I have lived. The middle version of the diet is Karl's preferred diet anyway, an amalgam of lean proteins, vegetables, and more "protein sachets" clocking in at a whopping twelve hundred calories a day. There are recipes in the back too, which all look very arcane and French.

Day 1

Karl says that when you are on a diet, "you are a general and you have a single soldier in your army. You must give him instructions and he must carry them out. It may annoy him but he has no choice." And thus I start the day with what Karl calls his "winter breakfast": a piece of toast, an egg (not fried in any oil, because that would be too appetizing), some juice, yogurt, and a Diet Coke. It is the spartan meal of a prisoner but it does the job.

After this, I decide to call my mother. I freely admit my mother is less fun than Karl Lagerfeld's mother. To wit—Karl Lagerfeld's mother told Karl he had "exceptionally ugly" hands and that he should never smoke. She also told him that his stories were "so boring" because he was six and that even though he was almost blind "children with glasses are the ugliest thing in the world," so she never bought him glasses. She was a great influence on Lagerfeld's life.

After my call, I set about guzzling Diet Cokes. Lagerfeld drinks up to ten Diet Cokes a day, so I have to really set my mind to this task. After three in quick succession I get very jittery; after four I decide I'm so jittery I can't eat lunch (protein sachet) or write or concentrate and just start pacing my room, which seems, all of a sudden, like a necessary activity. After my last Diet Coke, I give up and I go and watch the finale of *The Bachelor*. I rationalize this brainless but emotional activity because Karl is a rabid consumer of culture and has three hundred iPods. I have salmon with brussels sprouts for dinner and I am utterly starving afterward, although I feel so jittery. After the show finishes, I end up staying up until 7:00 a.m. reading about what Choupette does on the iPad. (She's a cat, so nothing.)

Day 2

Today I get up rather later than usual. I oversleep because I was reading so late, which Karl would never do. Karl sleeps exactly seven hours a night no matter what time he goes to bed. However, Karl also reads under a canopy in a room overlooking the Louvre and wears a white night shirt based on a seventeenth-century design he saw in the Victoria and Albert Museum. In penance, I decide to punish myself with Karl's "summer breakfast," which is even more barren than the "winter breakfast." (What is the point of seasonal menus for breakfast and breakfast only? I don't know.) It's just fruit and yogurt, basically. It is very hard not to have a second piece of toast, but Karl says, "The height of luxury is for me to have an extra slice of toast. It's the most delicious thing in the world." And now I agree with him.

For dinner, I make one of the dishes in the back of his diet book, "Veal with Plums," but there are no plums at the grocery store, so I make it with prunes. This is less good. I am starving for extra calories, so I have a glass of red wine. Dr. Dalí recommends two of those a day. A young doctor's notebook!

Day 3

Karl Lagerfeld does not usually like to entertain ("Lone-liness is a luxury for people like me," he has said), but he does have a recipe for quail flambé, which I have never had before. And can a woman just eat quail by herself? Apparently yes, because although I buy two quails (for $17; Karl is another one with an insane food budget), no one wants to eat them even though I ask in a plaintive voice. I have finally pushed my friends to the limit of their endurance, and quail is the last straw. It seems fitting. Karl says, "You have to be a real bore like me for the diet to work. When you are that boring, you have to make twice the effort in wit and conversation in order to com-pensate." But I really don't have the strength for that type of display this evening anyway.

If I am going to have quail flambé solo, the rest of the meal has to be, in some essential way, equally grandiose. This is what it means to be a dandy in modern society. I decide to make myself a traditional French multicourse meal using recipes from the Lagerfeld diet book. The first course is French onion soup. The onions are cooked with no butter whatsoever (usually, according to other recipes I have seen, the onions are cooked in an entire stick of but-ter); however, you are allowed to have a little Gruyère and croutons. Butter's absence makes the soup seem oddly flavorless, like onion soup I have had in a cafeteria. Still, it is not entirely off from the real thing.

Quail, however, is horrible. If you have never seen quail before (I hadn't), they are emaciated birds with dinosaur claws. If someone had ever grasped a quail in front of me and yelled, "This quail is rabid!" I would've believed them. I marinate the quail in wine for several hours. After a while, I take the quail out of the wine and then douse it in Grand Marnier and then set it on fire (flambé it). I don't have a match, so I light a paper towel on fire with the stove burner and then throw it on the quail. This works surprisingly well. The quail comes out tasting mostly of wine and burnt paper towel, but also of tiny shards of quail meat. The thing about quail is that it has absolutely no meat on it. It's only talons; that's it. I practically attack it with my teeth and I barely make a dent. I even have protein powder for dessert, I'm so hungry.

Day 4

I'm off the diet! I lost a couple of pounds and have managed to develop a sense of humor over the quail incident even though it was not funny at all at the time. As Karl says, "To follow a diet like this you have to have a sense of humor. Don't take things too seriously, make fun of yourself, admit why you're doing it. It's a physical thing, that's all. There's no point in pretending it's anything else."

And that really is the gift of Karl. So many celebrities try to pretend that they are dieting because of nutrition when actually they are dieting because they want to fit into a certain shape of clothing. Karl does not stand for such hypocrisy and even eats quail while he does it. And Choupette eats at the table with him (her own food, not quail).

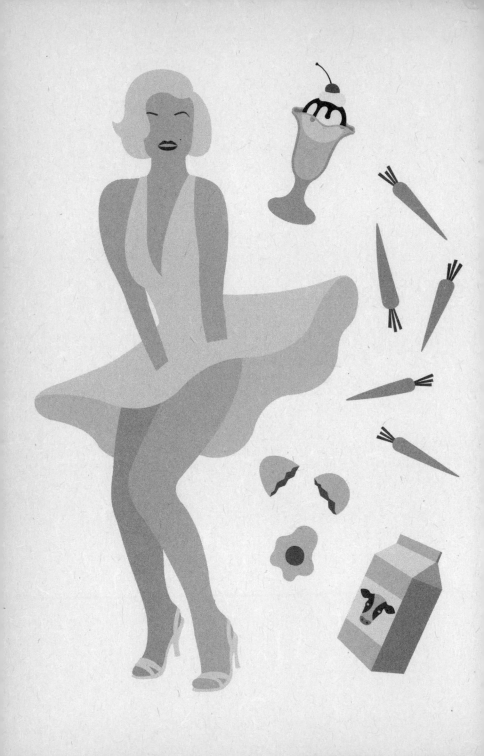

I Tried
Marilyn Monroe's Diet

In 1952, Marilyn Monroe gave an interview to the now-defunct *Pageant* magazine. To the gimlet eye of a serious journalist (not mine), it probably leaned too heavily on pictorials and subsections entitled "How to Feel Blonde All Over." But it did have something interesting to report: Marilyn Monroe's daily diet.

"I have been told my eating habits are absolutely bizarre," she confessed, right next to a picture of her dancing on an ottoman while wearing a Hawaiian shirt. "But I don't think so."

So, what were these famous habits? For breakfast, she would have two raw eggs whipped in warm milk: "I doubt any doctor could recommend a more nourishing breakfast for a working girl in a hurry." She would skip lunch, and then for dinner, she would broil liver, steak, or lamb and eat it with five carrots: "I must be part rabbit." And then she would have a hot-fudge sundae for dessert.

Does this sound insane or "bizarre" even? Maybe it does. But then, with the gimlet eye of a serious journalist, wasn't I duty-bound by the rules of my profession to try Marilyn's diet for myself and see if this was really true? Sure, I was. And in this spirit I decided to go forth and prosper. Besides, trying the diet of the sexiest woman in history could probably help me, and I definitely need help.

Preparation

My biggest worry with this diet is the raw eggs. How do you eat them and not get salmonella? To be safe, I go to Whole Foods and buy pasteurized eggs and discover that they are twice the price of normal eggs. I buy them anyway. I also go to the meat counter and ask if they have any liver. They do not. But they will have it in a few days. I make a note of it.

To dispel lingering worries, I call my grandmother. "Did you ever eat a raw egg?" I ask her. "No," she says. "But it will put hair on your chest." I nod into the phone.

Day 1

This morning, I start my diet. I am sort of excited but also full of dread, like Anne Hathaway before she hosted the Oscars. I take out the milk and heat it up in a saucepan. Once it is completely heated, I pour it, rather delicately, into a mug. Then I crack raw eggs into the mug and they plop into the milk, like two round globules of mucus. I stir them. The yolk comes apart in dribs and drabs, and the milk slowly turns yellow. It looks disgusting. I take one sip. To my surprise, it is utterly delicious! Like bland eggnog. I drink the whole thing in less than a minute. "Maybe this diet won't be too bad," I think to myself.

Not eating lunch, however, is incredibly hard, since I drank my eggs at 9:00 a.m. and am starving for the rest of the day. By 1:30 p.m., I could eat dinner, but I don't actually eat dinner until 8:00 p.m., when my friend and I feast on half a steak fillet and five raw carrots each. I am starving after dinner, as if I never ate it at all. Marilyn's life was extremely hard.

Day 2

On the second day, I wake up and know two things: I am hungry, and today is the day liver comes into Whole Foods. I am very excited because I have never had beef liver before. As I drink my egg milk, I imagine the liver awaiting me, quivering in its meat case. What should I do with it? Could it be good with ketchup?

After work, faint with hunger, I board a bus to the Whole Foods on Fifty-Seventh Street. I arrive, beaming, at the meat counter, where my request causes some confusion, nearly bringing me to tears in my fragile state. Eventually, a butcher emerges from the back room with several extremely bloody slabs of flesh. I immediately yip with joy and bring the liver back to my apartment. I wash the globs of blood off the liver and cook it. It is the worst thing I have ever had in my life. Such an odd taste, both bitter and meaty. I eat very little of it. In an effort to avoid waste, I chop it up and put it in the blender with a bunch of spices, old wine, and a stick of butter. I will make pâté, which I will save to reward myself when I complete the diet! It is very hard to pour the meat goo into a bowl and refrigerate it without eating it, but I do it.

Ravenous now, I go about making my sundae. Marilyn used to eat her sundaes at Wil Wright's ice-cream parlor, which is a California ice-cream producer known for its product's extremely high fat content. In the spirit of Marilyn's original sundae, I got the ice cream with the highest fat content and most natural ingredients I could find, a chocolate and a bourbon vanilla flavor. They are sort of horrible when mixed together. I eat it all, though.

Day 3

In order to do research for this project, I watch several Marilyn Monroe movies and discover an absolutely unwatchable farce costarring Yves Montand. Then I Google Marilyn Monroe's name and discover a cottage industry surrounding how to affect Marilyn Monroe's style and demeanor. There are a lot of forums and articles with tips like "Blink slowly" and "Use hormone cream to grow a downy hair on your face." One forum advocates smearing Vaseline all over your skin at night to moisturize it. Because I am crazy from lack of food, I do this. The next morning, my skin looks great! But I wonder how long this can last before my pores are completely clogged.

I am so hungry that I eat a lamb dinner at 3:00 p.m. I feel very tired and heavy. Can't tell if I am losing weight. I suspect this is a diet one can do only while also using recreational barbiturates.

Day 4

Today I am invited to a homemade-pizza party. This is a special kind of torture. I buy some ingredients and heroically eat nothing but a Baskin-Robbins sundae. When I leave and am standing in the subway terminal, I am so woozy I almost stumble onto the tracks. I can't sleep when I get home because my stomach hurts so badly. I think I need to get off this diet.

Day 5

After yesterday's spell, I take a break today so as not to die. I lie in my apartment the whole day recovering. I browse the Internet's vast network of Marilyn lifestyle websites and decide to start a different Monroe diet—the diuretic diet—tomorrow. Breakfast will be cereals and fruit juice. Lunch and dinner will be fish, diuretic vegetables, lots and lots of parsley, and the occasional "skimmed natural yogurt." It sounds like heaven in comparison.

Day 6

This diet is so much more humane. I have enough strength to do Marilyn's fitness regimen, which she described to *Pageant* as a "bust-firming routine." It requires you to lie on the ground holding weights above your head, then lift them and then hoist them in circles until you "feel tired." I can tell everyone at the gym thinks I look insane. I don't care. I almost die.

Days 7, 8, and 9

One Marilyn beauty tip that is actually kind of great is her emphasis on face highlighter. Much like pasteurized eggs, I never even knew this was a thing! I go to Sephora, buy some, and apply it next to my nose and between my eyebrows just like the forums say to. It absolutely covers up the huge pimples I sprouted from the Vaseline.

Day 10

Today is the last day of the diet. To celebrate, I sample my pâté. It tastes like decaying wine, but I put it on a cracker and eat it anyway. Yes, I have stayed basically the same weight and have a huge cystic pimple on my chin. But my breasts seem—slightly?—more firm, and I don't have to drink raw eggs anymore.

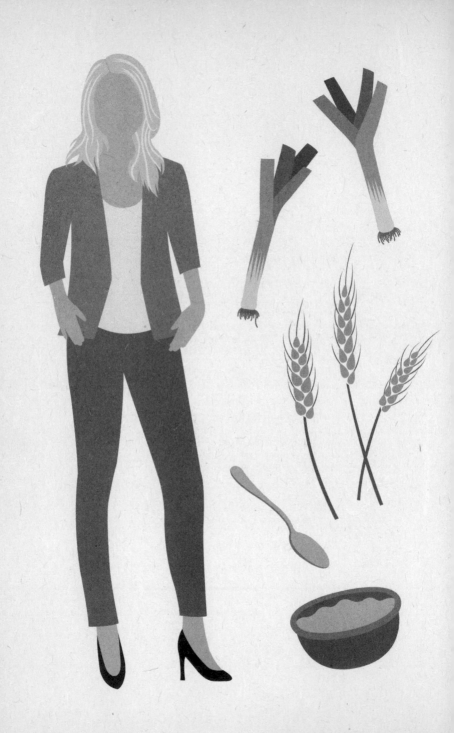

I Tried
Cameron Diaz's Diet

By her own admission, Cameron Diaz was one of those people who ate and ate and ate and never got fat. "I used to eat fried food from morning to night when I was in my twenties," she told *USA Today*. Then for some reason she began to feel that it wasn't "fair" to her body to keep eating with abandon, so she started eating much healthier foods that were stylish and tasteless, like quinoa and kale. For my part, I don't understand it. If I was skinny no matter what, I would eat a Burger King Rodeo Burger every day. But we are all different and special people, etc., etc.

In honor of her newly changed eating habits, Diaz wrote something called *The Body Book*, a kind of holistic nutrition manual that also apparently details Cam's diet and exercise routines. And unfortunately, where a new diet book emerges, I also am there, a kind of shadowy personage looking to capitalize on it! *Avanti*, dear readers!

Preparation

Preparation for this diet is pretty easy. Aside from actually buying the tome, I also decide to check out Cameron's press tour for *The Body Book*. I watch a particularly nervous appearance on *The Dr. Oz Show*. Cam says something nice about women being the most powerful force in the world and Dr. Oz sort of cackles derisively and then Cam spends most of the time on the show drinking water because apparently she drinks an entire glass when she wakes up every morning. It is very nerve-racking.

When I finally get the book in the mail, I realize it's rather less of a diet book, per se, and more of an *Our Bodies, Ourselves* experiment on how to be healthy. It has a long treatise on the skeleton and an even longer treatise on something Cameron calls the "lady body" that really is about getting your period. (How about we discuss something? No one should ever use the words "lady body" or "lady parts" or "lady problems" or "lady." There is enough horrible folksiness in America today without this particular branch of toothless feminist appropriation. It makes us sound so hokey. Never say "lady" again! It's "vagina"; Jesus Christ.) As a result, there is not much on her specific diet plan—it's more about the basic tenets of combining protein with carbohydrates and eating salmon for dinner and nuts as a snack. This is actually kind of nice—and certainly more normal for young impressionable "ladies" (No! Never!) to read about than a lot of these diet plans—but it leaves me in a bit of a spot. I have to delve into Cameron's nutrition another way. Her interviews! Unfortunately, one of the things I have to learn about Cameron is that her favorite meal is savory oatmeal. My lord, really?

Day 1

Today, I am trying to eat like Cameron before she became the healthy little *Goop*-let she is right now. I am going to revel in the old days, the salad days! The days of Justin Timberlake. I start the day off with a hearty breakfast— granola and a pancake—with my friend. This is not very Cameron, as she rarely ate breakfast in her younger years (a topic discussed in *The Body Book* at length), but whatever, I'm hungry.

After breakfast, I tuck in to watch the classic Cameron Diaz movie *The Counselor*. Have you seen *The Counselor*? I have never laughed harder at a movie before. It's a true ball of laughs. Is the movie about a drug deal? Who can say? At one point, Michael Fassbender utters the sentence "You have the most luscious lady body [not the term actually used] in all of Christendom," but he is not even the only person to use the word "Christendom" in the movie. Everyone uses it! Cameron Diaz plays a drug-dealing mastermind who owns a lot of cheetahs and they prowl around her pool.

After that, and now completely starving because I skipped lunch to watch *The Counselor* (I do not regret it), I decide to eat the most pre–health food–Cameron Diaz meal ever, the thing she ate every single day for two years after school. I go to a Mexican restaurant and order a bean burrito with extra cheese. I also get nachos. They are both extraordinarily delicious things, and I have no idea why she stopped eating like this.

Day 2

Now, unfortunately, I am going to have to start eating like the actual healthy Cameron Diaz. I suppose I had to eventually. I start the day with a huge glass of water. Apparently the first thing Cameron does when she wakes up is drink a huge glass of water just like she did on *The Dr. Oz Show*! This is because in the night you are "dehydrated simply from breathing." When Cameron drinks this water she goes "from being a wilted plant to one that has been rejuvenated by the rain." I go from a tired person to a person who is tired and whose stomach slightly hurts because it is filled with water. On to breakfast! One of Cameron's favorite breakfasts is "savory oatmeal," which is apparently oatmeal cooked "al dente, with caramelized leeks, green vegetables and ponzu sauce." Cameron describes it as "so good." I make the oatmeal and chop up a leek I bought and try to caramelize it (I burn it). I also realize my local grocery store doesn't sell ponzu sauce, so I make a version of it myself from a recipe I found online.

Finally, I combine the separate aspects together. You know what? It's weirdly delicious! The ponzu sauce is odd-tasting—it has a sweet and very citrusy flavor mixed with a faint soy aftertaste—but it does go well with the leeks.

Next, I go to the gym, because apparently Cameron is a workout fiend. Remember when she was dating A-Rod and she got so buff and then she fed him popcorn at the Super Bowl? They worked out together all the time.

I do a workout from her trainer that I found online and printed out beforehand. It's incredibly hard! You have to toss a medicine ball, do several lunges, and even deadlift something—a big, heavy bar in the style of a nineteenth-century bodybuilder. I don't have those kinds of muscles! I'm sore the rest of the day.

Day 3

Another day, another savory oatmeal, this time in "cake" form. It's another favorite breakfast of Cam's. I have to take a portion of yesterday's oatmeal and "sear it on high heat with a little olive oil" and then top it with egg whites. I thought this was going to be particularly bland, but it isn't that bad. It just seems like something a nineteenth-century bodybuilder would eat.

For lunch, I continue on the boring-food train with a recipe Cameron concocted of brown rice, lentils, quinoa, and kale mixed in a bowl. This may sound easy, but I screw it up terribly. I invite a friend to my apartment for lunch because audiences are really better for feats of spectacular healthfulness. After we talk for a while, I dump the rice and lentils into a pan and proudly leave the room to take a phone call. When I come back, the rice smells sort of awful, like it's burning. "Do you think the rice is burning?" my friend asks. "No," I say, and go over to check on the rice. It is burnt so badly I have to open a window, throw the rice in the trash, and take out the trash. Eventually, however, I remake the dish, and the end result is a bland bowl of rice with lentils. I do put Cholula Hot Sauce in it because Cameron is a big fan of Cholula Hot Sauce. My friend seems rather unimpressed by that.

Later, however, I am very productive at the gym. I deadlift far more weight than I did the day previous, and by that I mean I actually lift weights this time as opposed to just the bar.

For dinner for my final night of the Cameron diet, I decide to get Cuban food. It's Cameron's "ideal comfort food." I have shrimp tacos. They are unbelievably delicious, and again the magnitude of what Cameron gave up appears before me. How could she end all her years of eating delicious stuff for all this kale? Merely for muscle?

Still, you have to admire her; Cameron is trying (gamely) to be actually healthy and not propagate some odd gospel of weight loss. In fact, after the Cameron Diaz diet was over, I had actually gained weight, but I felt stronger and my skin was better. I guess life is all about small victories.

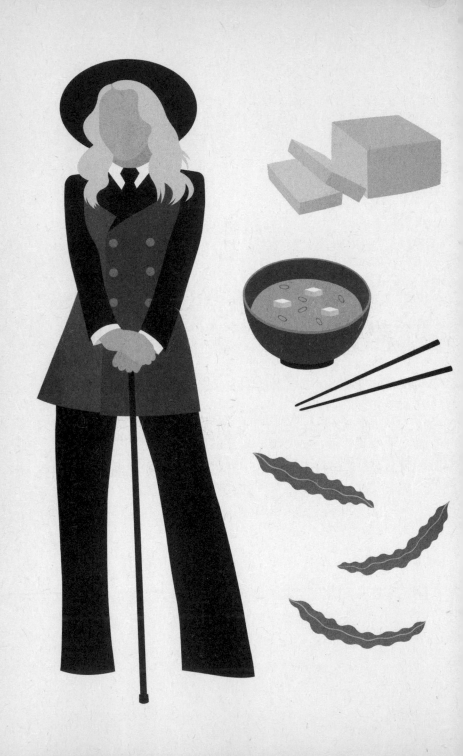

I Tried
Madonna's Diet

It has been exactly thirty years since Madonna exploded into the public consciousness with her debut album *Madonna,* and what great years they have been. Is there a woman out there more impressive than she is? Madonna is the top-selling female artist of all time. She has a son named Rocco. One time she was interviewed by Norman Mailer and he kept wanting to talk about feminism and its discontents and she subtly made fun of him the entire time and he did not seem to get it.

However, being Madonna is not easy. And how does she do it? She is fifty-six years old and she had to wear a crucifix on her butt at the Met Ball. Literally no one has ever done that before, and perhaps no one will ever do it again.

So, while Madonna's actual accomplishments are too much for the modern human to even contemplate, it would be nice to have her biceps at some point in my life. In that spirit, I decide to attempt Madonna's apparently draconian fitness and nutritional regimens. There is no time like the present to do something truly ambitious with your life.

Preparation

Madonna follows a very strict macrobiotic diet that abolishes the consumption of wheat, eggs, meat, and dairy and extols the benefits of something called "sea vegetables." You were expecting this woman to mess around? She does not mess around.

In order to follow Madonna's actual diet as closely as possible, I buy a cookbook written by Madonna's former private chef Mayumi Nishimura (who now is a sort of public apostle of macrobiotic living). It is called *Mayumi's Kitchen* and details various macrobiotic meals she used to serve Madonna and Madonna's starving passel of backup dancers. Madonna even wrote the foreword to the book. I am going to follow Mayumi's "10 Day Detox Diet." I hope it won't kill me. Some of the recipes, like "Tofu Tartar

Sauce" and "Sauerkraut with Thyme," sound a little suspect. I plan to do some of the recipes out of order for this
reason. I want to save the sauerkraut until the bitter end,
for example.

I also purchase Madonna's series of workout DVDs, as
one cannot be the queen of pop without a punishing fitness regimen. I am a little worried, because Madge is in
such good shape. Her trainer Nicole Winhoffer said she
has to put her in "really odd positions" before she even
feels an exercise. Madonna actually owns a series of gyms
in badass places like Moscow and Mexico City. They are
called Hard Candy Fitness. The DVD series is called
Addicted to Sweat, which I am not.

If I am going to be honest, this is altogether the strictest
diet veteran dieter Rebecca Harrington has undertaken.
Will it be horrible? Or will it be as awesome as the time
Madonna eviscerated Mike Myers in *Interview* magazine? (Madonna: "Would you ask me some questions
that have a resonance to my life? This interview is mostly
about what you're interested in: toys and hockey.") I simply don't know.

Day 1

I start the day with a nourishing portion of miso soup and brown rice. I was worried I would not have the stomach for miso soup in the morning, but I really enjoy it and it's rather filling. It's so filling that I skip lunch and don't eat until dinnertime, which is a stew of barley and seaweed. It is not very good, and I sort of regret that I missed out on the soy meat and spiral rice pasta of lunch. But do you think Madonna engages in regrets of this nature? This is a woman who wrote a song where the chorus goes "I'm not your bitch / Don't hang your shit on me." In the background of this chorus, she whispers, "Handle it." So, no, I don't think she would.

Day 2

In order to give your "stomach a break" from the tremendous strain of sea-vegetable barley stew, Mayumi suggests that you start off day 2 with a heaping portion of steamed greens and a Fuji apple. I am getting a little hungry now, I must admit. I am seeing the puritanical nature of this diet. A woman cannot survive on greens alone.

I keep wandering around New York City listening to "Papa Don't Preach" to take my mind off my all-encompassing hunger, and it strikes me how revolutionary Madonna was. Did you know that Madonna dedicated that song to the pope because she hated "male authorities"? And the pope is called "*il Papa*" in Italian! (Clever!) I mean, what pop star even cares about standing up to the pope now? Or male authorities? Pop stars today are just like, "Male authorities, how am I doing? Am I the prettiest? You tell me!" or "Where is the pope? Is he on a bus? I am going to visit him!"

Day 3

Today I decide to do my first *Addicted to Sweat* DVD. I am so scared. On the outside it has a massive picture of Madonna, like Stalin in Moscow, looking beautiful and addicted to sweat. She is presiding over a tiny graphic of a woman (it's Nicole, Madonna's personal trainer, I find out later) doing an insane move where she holds the back of her foot near her head. When I actually put the DVD on, it does not mention Madonna, play her music, or feature her in any way. The whole workout stars Nicole in what seems to be a Russian warehouse doing incomprehensibly difficult dance moves. She keeps jumping, and there are a lot of "ball changes" going on. Madonna is only implied. Handle it!

Later that day, I make something called tofu tartar sauce, which is just tremendously disgusting and lumpier than it should be because I do not have a strainer.

Day 4

One time Madonna told *Spin*'s Bob Guccione Jr. that "straight men only think about how you may dominate them in some way and make their dicks shrivel up or something." In that aggressive yet very fun spirit, I start my day off with corn in a plum-paste sauce. It is good, actually. It gives me a sugar rush because I have not had sugar for several days, even in plum-covered-corn form.

Days 5 and 6

Madonna, at least in her younger years, took time off from her rigorous dieting schedule on the weekends and ate whatever she wanted. In honor of her, I do the same, but the truth is, I am basically dying on this diet. I don't know how Madonna lives. It is so hard to give up all those foods. Literally every food! It is not Mayumi's fault. She is doing the best she can with tofu tartar sauce, but there is just not all that much you can do.

Day 7

Back on the diet, I have to make tofu cheese for a quinoa salad I will consume in three days. Why do I have to
make this cheese now? Because the tofu has to be spread
with miso and kept in a sealed container for three days so
that it rots a little, not unlike cheese! Spreading this tofu
with miso is actually hard. I am so hungry I eat a little of
the raw miso.

Later, I decide to go out to (macrobiotic!) dinner with a
friend who notices I keep really cleaning my plate on this
diet in a compulsive way I never do normally. "It's like you
are starving!" he says. I feel like I am starving, but I am
definitely not. I am eating food. I am just hungrier than
I have ever been. I mean, as old Madge once said, "How
can you be *like* a virgin?" So how could it be *like* I am
starving? I am not actually starving, I don't think.

Day 8

Today, I decide to have a macrobiotic dinner party. I
invite all my usual friends, who seem decidedly unhappy
about this new theme. I make Mayumi's sweet-and-sour
tempeh and brown rice with almonds on it, with a side of

sauerkraut. Guess what? Everyone loves the sauerkraut, which I bought from a store. It is universally acclaimed as the best dish there.

Days 9 and 10

It is the end of the diet! And in celebration I do my last *Addicted to Sweat* DVD, called *Jaw Breaker Chair: Dripping Wet*. I was so scared of this DVD the whole week that I actually hid it in my couch. Finally, I find it in my couch and play it. It is so hard! It involves doing push-ups with your feet on a chair.

I saved the tofu cheese for my last meal on the diet. It has been rotting in my fridge relatively unmolested for three days and now it is time for its moment in the sun. I combine the tofu cheese with quinoa to make a gross salad. The tofu cheese tastes surprisingly like tofu, yet combined with quinoa it has an odd granularity. I am supposed to finish the diet with a tofu scramble, but I can't even do it. I have some fried chicken instead.

So, in conclusion, is Madonna's diet hard? You bet your ass it is. Is it fun? No! Do you have to eat sauerkraut?

Yes! But what I really realized is that Madonna is a feminist revolutionary and it's hard to be on a revolutionary's diet. She danced in a wedding dress! She called David Mamet a chauvinist! She made a sex book called *Sex*! Paul McCartney may have suspiciously brown hair, but no one says he tries too hard to be young! I guess the question is this: Did Susan B. Anthony eat sauerkraut every day? Probably she did.

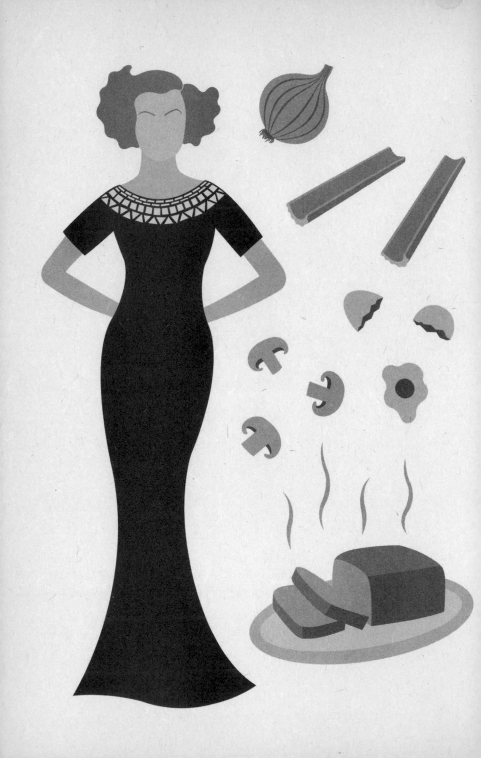

I Tried
Greta Garbo's Diet

In the thirties, famously reclusive actress Greta Garbo met self-described "doctor of natural science" (i.e., doctor of nothing) Gayelord Hauser, nutritionist to the stars. They reportedly hit it off, which is saying a lot, because Garbo had very few friends, hated going out, and once refrained from speaking a single word during a dinner with Mae West.

But Garbo and Hauser were bonded by their love of calorie restriction. Garbo had begun shedding pounds in 1924, after Louis B. Mayer told her, "In America, men don't like fat women," and she dieted continuously throughout her life. She particularly loved fad diets, which made her a good disciple for Hauser's science; he had written several books about nutrition, including *New Health Cookery* and his most famous tome, *Look Younger, Live Longer*, in which he suggested eating raw yeast and drinking buttermilk as a fun treat.

Garbo was an adherent of the Hauser regimen, which emphasized the glories of vegetables, nuts, and yogurt, for many years. Some publications even speculated that the two were having an affair based around their shared love of disgusting food. They often cohabitated, and a neighbor of theirs in Palm Beach once complained of their exploits, writing, "that skinny Swedish actress and her fancy boyfriend are always running around naked in their backyard." Though Simon Doonan described Garbo as Hauser's "longtime beard." Whether they had an affair or not, here was a chronic dieter who lived with her nutritionist. Garbo was living the dream! So I wanted to emulate that in some small, sad, yet thoroughly modern way for my latest experiment in historically validated strange eating habits.

Preparation

After a rather exhaustive search, I find two of Hauser's aforementioned books on the Internet and buy them.

When I finally receive the books in the mail, they're quite dusty and a little intimidating. Neither seems to have been opened since they were published in 1930 and 1951; when I crack the spine of one, I start sneezing.

The first line to *Look Younger, Live Longer* is "You are making a mistake." Why? Because you are treating this book "like any other book" when it is in fact "a passport for a new way of living."

Hauser believes that if you fuel your body with "wonder foods" you can live until you are one hundred. In case you are curious, wonder foods are: brewer's yeast, wheat germ, and molasses, apparently all rich in various vitamins and minerals that will guarantee long life. These are not easy products to procure in the modern world. Edible yeast is quite hard to find (the stuff that makes bread rise is not something you can just pop in your mouth) and looks very disgusting and inedible when I buy a version you can sprinkle on cereal at a health food store next to my apartment. Apparently yeast is quite nutritious. My grandmother tells me that she had a relative who used to eat yeast all the time. "Of course she did have stomach troubles," she tells me.

The recipes in both books look absolutely terrifying. There is one particularly horrible-looking one for a "celery loaf," which Hauser defends as "really delicious" and consists of pureed celery, nuts, and milk. There is something about this combination that makes me involuntarily shudder. Luckily, I also find an exhaustive fan website devoted to Garbo's eating habits. Apparently she loved dried apricots.

Day 1

In one of Garbo's first and only interviews, she told a reporter in exasperation, "I was born. I had a mother and father. I went to school. What does it matter?" It is in that spirit of Lutheran simplicity that I start my diet with one of Garbo's favorite lunches: "a cup of chicken broth with chives, cottage cheese, half a ripe avocado with a vinegar, herb and oil dressing, a slice of pineapple and one piece of toasted and buttered dark bread." Although this dizzying array of food does not go together in the classic sense, it is not exactly terrible. It is just plain. Terrible comes with dinner, which is based on Hauser's meal for Garbo the first night he met her: a veggie burger "consisting of wild rice and chopped hazelnuts, mixed with an egg and fried in soybean oil," plus a dessert of "a broiled grapefruit with [blackstrap] molasses in the center!" The veggie burgers take a long time to cook and taste predominantly of eggs.

The hazelnuts are an unpleasant surprise. Broiled grape-fruit tastes medicinal. I am not very hungry, just confused about why these ingredients have been paired together.

Day 2

There was a period in Garbo's life where she subsisted almost entirely on "chicken, dried apricots and whole milk, with brown beans and biscuits for snacks." This is actually a fun day. Whole milk is delicious, and brown beans are very filling. I eat chicken I bake in the oven. I feel like I am in the army in 1942.

Garbo retired from acting at the age of thirty-six after she appeared in the notorious flop *Two-Faced Woman*. (This is a crazy movie in which Garbo plays fake twin sisters and has to dance for a very long time. She is not a good dancer.) Soon thereafter she moved to New York and did most of her grocery shopping about ten blocks away from my apartment. I could have bought apricots at the same store she did! I feel like we were practically neighbors, except she lived in a beautiful castle on the East River and I do not.

Day 3

Garbo was born Greta Lovisa Gustafsson in Stockholm in 1905. Although she got rid of her original name, she always said she "missed" the food of her native Sweden. She once brought what was probably lingonberry jam to Italy and flummoxed the Italians when she put it on her cornflakes and then poured coffee over it. In honor of Garbo's affinity for her own country's cultural heritage, I eat waffles with lingonberry jam on them. Then Swedish meatballs with lingonberry jam on them. It's delicious!

Day 4

Back on the Hauser regimen, I start the day with his notorious "pep breakfast"—two raw eggs beaten in orange juice. Hauser describes it as a "creamy drink fit for a King's table." I do not feel the same way. This is so much worse than the raw eggs in milk that I drank for the Marilyn Monroe diet. If pneumonia were a food, this is what it would taste like.

Later, I go to a bar with some friends. Garbo enjoyed the occasional drink, even in the depths of a diet. When she transitioned to the talkies, her first line on-screen was,

"Gimme a whiskey, ginger ale on the side, and don't be stingy, baby!" That is an awesome thing to say, but I don't say it. I have a hamburger, a Hauser favorite, but I am still hungry. I also drink a beer.

Day 5

Today is a special day. It is the day I will finally make the thing that has been ruining my life since I first heard about it: the celery loaf. Around 4:00 p.m., I psych myself up to do it. I puree the celery in my blender until it is a green mush. Then I add walnuts, parsley, onions, mushrooms, butter, eggs, and bread crumbs. The whole thing becomes an awful brown goop. I pour this into a baking dish and cover it with a lot of milk. Then I bake it. While it bakes, it smells like a rotting body. Finally, after thirty minutes, it is ready. Now, I am no baby. I have gladly eaten peanut butter with steak. I drank raw eggs in milk for several days. I even had tofu cheese.

Yet, when I open up my oven to get out my celery loaf, I start to dry-heave. It smells like I just put vomit in a baking pan and baked it for thirty minutes. I slam the oven door shut, spray the entire place with Lysol, and leave my apartment.

Day 6

Today is the day of the Oscars. (Greta Garbo never won one! She just got an honorary one.) The people I invited over to watch the Oscars are eating popcorn and sushi. I am eating this weird Hauser recipe for "Swiss Steak," which is steak you dip in bread crumbs, fry, and then boil in water. It is incredibly soggy and bland, and I am so hungry. Sometimes, I see the celery loaf peering at me from inside the oven, since I haven't cleaned it out yet. My guests ask me what is in there. Maybe they can smell it.

Days 7 and 8

In the next two days, I devote myself to "wonder foods." I follow Hauser's reducing plan, which has me drinking buttermilk with yeast (this tastes like yogurt mixed with something oddly breadlike and mealy), milk with molasses and yeast (this tastes like the worst milk shake of all time), and wheat germ on cereal (wheat germ tastes like quinine). For dinner, I have hamburger patties and liver. Liver, which used to disgust me, might be delicious. This diet might have broken me. It reminds me of the time Garbo just didn't even go to her own wedding. She was probably overwhelmed.

Day 9

I attempt the first diet Garbo ever tried. According to legend, Garbo ate nothing but spinach for three weeks to lose the weight Louis B. Mayer told her to lose. I am sort of relieved I don't have to eat weird substances anymore, but I am really starving and it is extremely hard to eat only spinach when you already have been dieting for a while and there is a celery loaf that is still in your oven. But Garbo had tremendous willpower. Once on a trip to Italy, her lunch consisted only of yellow and red carrots, which she insisted had different flavors. I use that mental image as my guide, waiting until lunch to eat, when I have a big bowl of raw spinach. For dinner, I have sautéed spinach. After dinner, I take a walk. Garbo loved walks and used to walk from her apartment on Fifty-Second Street to Washington Square Park and then back. I meet my friend in the West Village. I am so hungry that I sort of cheat at her apartment and eat some dried fruit and a spoonful of gelato. But what is a spoonful of gelato when you are already in such a deep dark hole?

Day 10

I am off the diet! I lost four pounds officially and look rather ill. (I am pale, and my cheeks are unusually prominent.) But I have a great respect for the grande dame of movie acting. No wonder she "want[ed] to be alone." She had to bear the pain of such an insane eating regimen without the impertinent attention of the world.

Several days after the diet has finished and I am eating normally again, I return home to my apartment and smell something awful. It is the heart of darkness/my celery loaf, and it is still in my oven.

I forgot about it, but the time has come to confront my demon in its celery face. I take it out of the oven; the smell of rotting celery is overpowering and immediately I gag. I put it on the counter. I take a small piece, eat it, and then promptly scoop the whole loaf into a small trash bag. I need a whiskey.

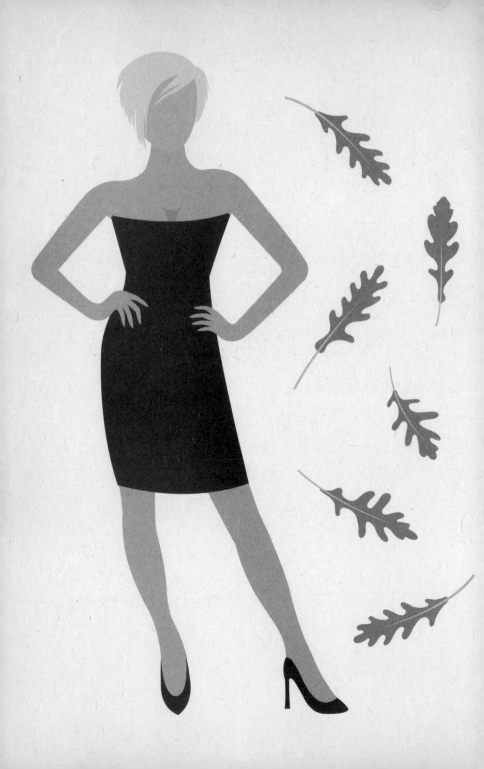

I Tried
Victoria Beckham's Diet

Victoria Adams, a.k.a. Posh Spice, a.k.a. Victoria Beckham, is known not only for her nonverbal tenure with the Spice Girls and her eventual ascension to the perch of successful fashion designer but also for her tremendously svelte frame, which has survived several pregnancies unscathed. She once told an interviewer, "I'm not going to lie—I'm not one of those people that says, 'Oh, I eat hamburgers.'" It is nice that she is honest in a world of liars, although a woman who wrote a 528-page autobiography when she was only twenty-seven probably does not have a problem with honesty. I actually read this autobiography and I loved it! It chronicled the whole story of her life and ended with a whodunit mystery. Even Mark Twain couldn't do that.

Even though I am now almost woefully experienced at dieting, I am slightly nervous about trying Victoria's various diets. Beckham is known for her commitment to dieting. One time, at a restaurant, she ate only arugula, and it didn't even have any dressing on it. Can mere mortals do what she does to stay skinny?

Preparation

In recent years, Posh has publicized her diets, reportedly following the Five Hands Diet after her daughter, Harper, was born and later tweeting about the Honestly Healthy alkaline diet. I plan to follow all of these regimens, although I do not have Victoria's stamina, willpower, or ability to just pose while other people are singing.

Day 1

The Five Hands Diet is exactly what it sounds like. You eat only five handfuls of food in a day and then for some unknown reason you declare yourself full. A fun surprise about this diet is that the portion is not even really the size of a hand. It is actually the size of a palm. The five hands (palms) of food have to be protein. Of course, you can have as many vegetables as you want. (But who cares? You can always have that on every diet. It seems a hollow gesture.)

I start the day off with two eggs. They are small eggs because they have to fit in my palm. It's not a terrible breakfast, but it is a terrifying breakfast, because I realize how little a palm actually holds. I know I do not have the self-control of Victoria. I didn't have a fruit plate instead of a cake for my birthday like she did in 2012. (Although one time Victoria's mom made her a cake in the shape of a fruit plate. There is a picture of it in her autobiography.)

After my eggs, I go to the gym. Early on in her career, Victoria said she never went to the gym and hated it. She even posed the question "What do you wear on the running machine?" because she never wore flat shoes. But at some point during her tenure in Los Angeles she decided to start running. Now apparently she cycles in an egg pod to prevent cellulite. This is what America does to people.

So now that Victoria is all into running, I suppose I'll try it too (especially because where did she find an egg pod to ride a bike in?). I go to my gym (an oft-forgotten friend) and try my hand at the treadmill. Running is really rather difficult. All the bouncing makes for poor TV watching. I last only ten minutes and quickly exit.

After the gym, I decide to eat a small hand-size portion of a protein-based kale smoothie. (This is hard to measure, but I think I do a good job.) This does not fill me. In an hour I have a palm-size portion of a protein bar. I feel an odd sense of panic.

Another thing to know about Posh is that she has actually written not one but two books! In 2006, Posh followed up her autobiography with a book called *That Extra Half an Inch*—a 384-page fashion advice book. (The woman writes in an expansive style.) I suppose it's a bit dated now. For example, Victoria says, "One thing I really love is a starchy tulle skirt. They can really prettify an outfit." She also recommends bringing lacquered beads and velvet opera gloves to a party.

But anyway, in the book, she confesses to wearing fake nails (and fake toenails!). And at around 4:00 p.m., in my most desperate moment on the Five Hands Diet, I consider getting very long fake nails like Howard Hughes just so my hand will be slightly longer and therefore able to accommodate more food. And then I remember that this is really the palm diet. Nails don't matter. And I sob on the street.

I know that other people graze all day and it doesn't affect them in the least, and they feel energized and fulfilled. I, definitively, do not. I need big, serious meals to feel complete, like Henry VIII. I am dying when I have my last snack of almonds at 4:00 p.m., and when I finally eat at 9:00 p.m., I eat far more than the handful of sashimi I thought I was going to eat. I end up eating an actual hand of sushi. With nails!

Day 2

Victoria Beckham actually tweeted about the alkaline diet relatively recently, and I took it upon myself to find out what that was all about. Usually VB (which is how she signs her Twitter) tweets about her new collection or a "vintage" Spice Girls pizza that has been frozen in her fridge for ten years, so I am assuming this diet is important. I bought the book VB recommends, called *Eating the Alkaline Way*. It's a really nice-looking cookbook; it even has a vegetable mini-pizza on the front!

Eating the Alkaline Way is based on the idea that you should be eating "alkaline" foods, a.k.a. foods that are not acidic. Luckily, acidic foods happen to be all fats, all meats, all eggs, and most carbohydrates. What a coincidence! It seems to me like a way to cut out all fat by pretending that fat is acid. For example, *lemons* are alkaline? I mean, that makes as much sense as the lyrics to "Spice Up Your Life."

My first day on the alkaline diet starts out rather well. I begin the day with a bok choy shake and quinoa-flake porridge with homemade macadamia nut milk and pomegranate seeds. The bok choy shake is whatever (the green drinks are just turning into one long blur at this point), but the porridge is actually absolutely delicious. I love macadamia nut milk! It tastes almost as good as real milk. And the porridge tastes a bit like porridge. Victory in our time.

The problem with flying to great heights is that like the Spice Girls, you think you can do anything. Sponsor a frozen pizza. Call an album *Schizophonic*. Get really long extensions with one nonmatching streak in them. Guess what? You can't. You can't do any of that. Just because you're in the Spice Girls doesn't mean that all is permitted. You're going to fall back to earth eventually.

I experience the fallout from this sort of hubris when I decide to make the falafel in *Eating the Alkaline Way*. I am flying so high from the whole nut-milk thing, and it actually doesn't even bother me at first that this falafel is made entirely of seeds and held together by carrots. I just mosey along, like Victoria starting a jeans collection. I realize something is amiss after I grind up all the seeds and the carrots in a blender and try to make falafel-style balls with them. Here is a tip for your future: You cannot make seeds into balls. You just can't. Even if you bake them at very low heat, like they say to in *Eating the Alkaline Way* (which is starting to sound like a spiritual text!). It's simply impossible. I eat a couple of the seeds, but after a while I just give up.

After lunch, I decide to have dinner, which is soybean broth with a bunch of vegetables in it. It is terrible and I throw out most of it. I'm exhausted and hungry, and the food was so disgusting today I realize I didn't even eat five hands of food. I ate, like, three hands. Posh, how do you do it?

Day 3

Day 3 starts with a relatively normal breakfast of avocado toast. I usually find that a hearty breakfast, but I'm absolutely starving when I eat it. Maybe I like acid?

Finally, I go to lunch in the Meatpacking District, in anticipation of VB's first store, which will be opening up there in the fall. When you think about it, it is kind of amazing that Posh has transformed her life to this degree. She went from a soccer wife to a phenomenally successful fashion designer. You could tell from the nascent days of the Spice Girls that she is obsessed with clothing. There is a harrowing scene in her autobiography where she sleeps in Gianni Versace's bed and Naomi Campbell is mean to her.

Anyway, in order to celebrate Victoria's becoming the woman she wanted to become, I am going to order the "girlie" lunch menu she planned for her *Vogue* interview ("no tomatoes in the salad, balsamic vinegar instead of vinaigrette, a Diet Coke"), but at the last minute I order chicken. Even though chicken is an acidic food! The diet has come to an end.

After my travails are finished, for "research" I actually watch the movie *Spice World*. I used to think that was such a boring movie when I was little (my sister loved it). The problem was, I totally didn't get it at the time. It's actually a genius satire on the concentric circles of fame and capitalism in Cool Britannia—even a metatextual comment on how ridiculous a "Spice Girls movie" is as a thing. Essentially, it's in on its own joke. And Victoria Beckham is too. As she says, "I'm so camp! I'm such a gay man trying to get out. I don't give a f**k what anybody thinks!"

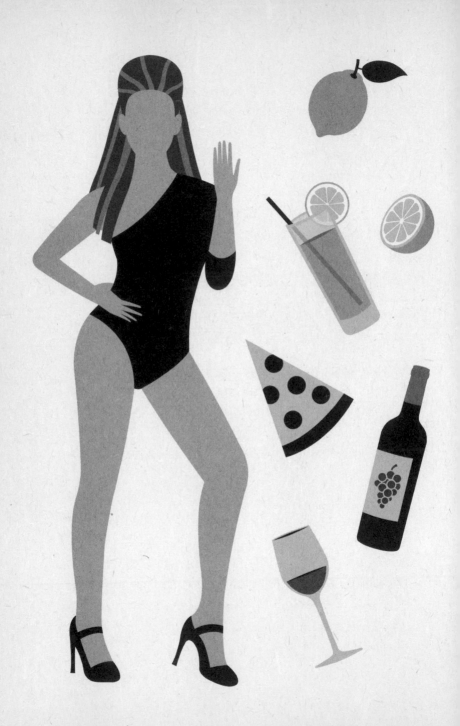

I Tried
Beyoncé's Diet

I have seen Beyoncé's HBO documentary, *Life Is But a Dream*, a startling number of times. There are so many parts I like: When Beyoncé brings her computer into an elevator and films herself in the elevator. When Beyoncé talks to a mysterious man off-camera who is wearing glasses. When Beyoncé says, "Life is but a dream!" to Jay Z and Feist is playing in the background. I could go on.

But my favorite part of all is when Beyoncé prepares for her performance at the 2011 Billboard Music Awards. At first, it looks like the whole thing is going to be a disaster. The rehearsal space gets screwed up. The special effects guys are worried about the army of digital Beyoncés they are making out of computers. Beyoncé has to coordinate her dancing with the digital Beyoncés, which is difficult. Finally, Beyoncé does a video diary. Only one eye is shown on-camera, and the other eye is off-camera for some reason. Beyoncé talks about throwing in the towel and giving up. She can accept defeat when she is defeated, she says. You think it's all over. Then the next scene is the most amazing performance I have ever seen a human do.

This is the thing about Beyoncé: She has the best baby, and she gives performances normal people couldn't ever do even with ten years of rehearsal time. Naturally, her fitness and dieting regimens are things mere mortals can barely contemplate. As a professional dieter, I have to do her various diets before I die. But will my attempting Beyoncé's lifestyle be a hard-luck story that ultimately pays off with amazing success, like Beyoncé at the Billboard Music Awards? Or just a regular hard-luck story, which usually ends in failure?

Preparation

One thing I have always enjoyed about Beyoncé is that she's very open about how hard it is to eat like she does. This is refreshing, as most celebrities are always saying crazy things like, "I eat pizza but I eat it moderately." One time Beyoncé called herself "a natural fat person, just dying to get out."

I have decided to do the entire range of Beyoncé's diets. I will endure the Master Cleanse, which Beyoncé endured when she lost weight for *Dreamgirls*; I will attempt the Herculean diet Beyoncé used to lose weight after birthing Blue Ivy. I will subject myself to Beyoncé's daily fitness and nutritional travails. I mean, this is a woman who, in 2005, hired someone to film her for sixteen hours a day. She knows how to look good.

Days 1 and 2

MASTER CLEANSE

Beyoncé was apparently inspired by Tom Hanks, who lost fifty pounds for his role in *Cast Away*, when she decided to lose twenty pounds for her part in *Dreamgirls*. To do it, she decided to use the Master Cleanse, a diet first developed in the forties that involves consuming only lemonade made out of cayenne pepper, lemons, and grade-B maple syrup (do *not* get grade A, in the Lord's name) nine times a day. You can't eat food. You also have to consume something called the Salt Water Flush (salt water that you drink while looking at yourself in the mirror, according to a forum on the subject) that is supposed to "help" your digestive tract.

Now, as a veteran dieter, I have done the Master Cleanse before. Of course I have! It was all the rage in 2006 because of Beyoncé. I have to say, the first time I tried it, I did not love it. I lasted only a day or two. One of my big problems was that I didn't understand the Salt Water Flush. This time, however, in the name of journalistic integrity, I have decided I will try the Master Cleanse in a real way. Just like Tom Hanks did for *Cast Away*.

So, bright and early on a spectacularly gray Monday, I get all the ingredients at the grocery store and set about making my lemonade. It's hard to squeeze the lemons by hand (I have very weak arms), but the lemonade itself is not bad. It tastes like a spicier version of regular lemonade. For the first couple of hours I'm on the diet, it's fine. The spiciness of the lemonade mitigates my hunger throughout the morning. By 3:00 p.m., however, my stomach starts to feel the effect of food deprivation. It is hard to have lemonade for dinner. I don't recommend it.

Later, I go to a vaudevillian revue in a basement. While I'm watching a man put on a surgical gown and sing a humorous song about being a doctor, I think about how Beyoncé said she felt "cranky" on the Master Cleanse because other people on the *Dreamgirls* set were eating Krispy Kremes near her. The one good thing about this vaudeville revue is that they don't serve Krispy Kremes at all, just Shirley Temples with vodka in them. But even those are making me so hungry I eventually have to leave.

The next day, however, something odd happens. I'm way less hungry than I was the day before. I actually look forward to my spicy lemonade, as if it were an old friend. I don't even really care when people eat food near me. Has the Master Cleanse rid me of the need for solid food? It is a question.

Day 3

THE MASTER CLEANSE WITHOUT QUALITIES

I'm moving out of my tiny midtown garret (to a location unknown! I still do not have an apartment), but this does not stop me from Master Cleansing. At this point, I have completely conquered hunger. I feel like an eleven-year-old

Beyoncé running a punishing rehearsal with an early version of Destiny's Child. I don't even want solid food. I offer my movers Master Cleanse lemonade, but they say no.

I go to Dunkin' Donuts to get doughnuts for the movers and I force myself to have a tiny piece of a doughnut. It's actually a little scary. I've lost four pounds in the space of three days.

Day 4

CHEAT DAY

Off the Master Cleanse, but still not particularly hungry, I decide to embark on Beyoncé's cheat day. Apparently once a week, Beyoncé consumes "pizza and wine." In solidarity with B, I decide to have that exact same meal. I regain my appetite after eating the first piece of pizza. I end up eating four pieces.

Days 5 and 6

Beyoncé has a very extensive tour rider. One time, she requested red toilet paper. She also asks for "oatcakes," which resemble a dry tea biscuit in which oats play a prominent role. While apple picking with my friends in upstate New York, I nosh on the aforementioned oatcakes while my friends eat delicious bread and cheese. Oatcakes aren't bad, but they aren't very filling in comparison.

Later, my friends take several photos of me eating an apple and put them on Instagram. If I had been Beyoncé, I would have demanded they take them down, but as it is I'm too scared.

Days 7 and 8

For the next two days, I'm doing what is probably the hardest part of all Beyoncé's diets: the post-pregnancy eating plan that allowed her to lose sixty pounds in three months.

This particular diet is very rich in protein, like most good diets in vogue today. You start the day with egg whites, consume slices of turkey with capers for lunch, eat cucumbers with vinegar and lemon for snacks, and finish the day with yellowtail sashimi with jalapeños and wasabi. Sometimes you are allowed to have frozen yogurt.

I have to say, the actual food on this diet is not terrible. It's sparse, yes, but flavorful. If I were not slowly going broke from ordering all that yellowtail sashimi at my local sushi place, it would generally be fine.

The real hardship of this particular regimen is the exercise. Beyoncé worked out for two hours a day to get rid of her baby weight, and it is hard for a working woman with a busy schedule of going to vaudeville revues to find the time for that. I end up splitting the workouts into an hour-long strength-training routine and an hour-long run. It's Beyoncé's music that gets me through it. I keep listening to the song "Run the World (Girls)," but in my head I change the lyrics to keep me motivated. "If women really ran the world (girls!) I would not be running for two hours. LOL! They don't run anything!" Har har har. Whatever, working out for two hours is lonely.

Day 9

Today, I eat the "Sasha Salad," a favorite salad of Beyoncé's, based, I imagine, on her former alter ego Sasha Fierce. (Beyoncé eventually killed her.) It is a chicken salad with jalapeños in it. It's okay. For research, I looked up "Sasha Fierce" on Wiki Answers, and they define her as a "sociable" twenties singer famous for "curing the Great Dpression [*sic*] in America" and working at the post office.

Day 10

The diet is completed! (Run the world, girls!) And I feel like a new woman. This is the most effective regimen I have ever undertaken. Between the Master Cleanse and Beyoncé's post-pregnancy diet, I have lost ten pounds. I never lost this much weight, even while eating the protein sachets of Karl Lagerfeld. Beyoncé is really good at life.

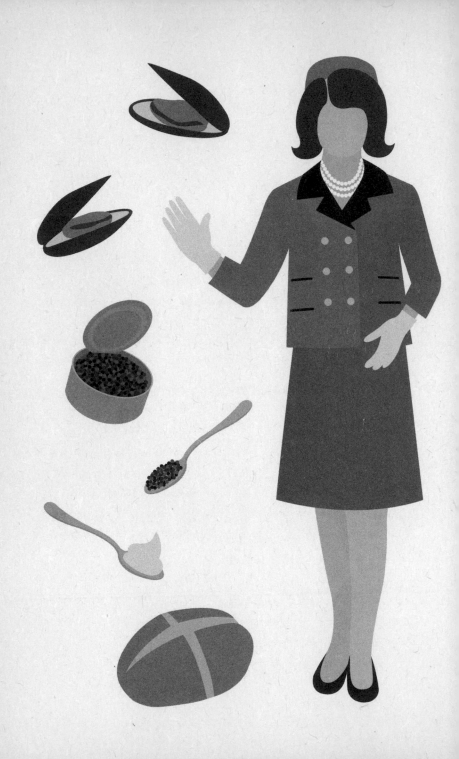

I Tried
Jackie Kennedy's Diet

When you are from New England, certain truths are indisputable. Iced coffee is a seasonless beverage; whimsical bow ties are appropriate for family parties. And the Kennedy family is important and their dramas are absorbing.

Thus, it was with reverence and the inborn curiosity of a New Englander that I decided to become "a Jackie" for my latest diet experiment. Jackie has always been my favorite Kennedy, for her ability to speak French and the time when she reportedly declared: "Why worry if you're not as good at tennis as Eunice or Ethel, when men are attracted by the feminine way you play tennis?" That is a sentiment with which I wholeheartedly agree.

Jackie Kennedy famously watched her weight "with the rigor of a diamond merchant counting his carats," according to one poetic staff member. One diet consisted, according to legend, of nothing but a single baked potato, stuffed with beluga caviar and sour cream, eaten once a day. Since that diet is exorbitantly expensive and vaguely insane, I decide to bolster my Jackie Kennedy diet with recipes and practices from her housekeeper Marta Sgubin's cookbook, *Cooking for Madam*.

Preparation

Caviar is a surprisingly difficult thing to buy. For example, you cannot just go to Gristedes and demand caviar, because I have tried it. I decide to purchase my caviar at the Grand Central Terminal fish market in midtown. I am initially shocked (and rather outraged) that the tiny amount I'm buying costs approximately thirty dollars. By comparison, though, this is cheap. Jackie Kennedy's favorite type of caviar, beluga, comes from a sturgeon found in the seas of the former Soviet Union. According to Wikipedia, it retails for approximately $7,000 to $10,000 per kilogram. It was even illegal for a while in 2005, and you cannot eat it with a metal spoon. You have to eat it with a mother-of-pearl spoon. I decide that once again, I must sacrifice my art in the face of practical reality. "This is like *New Grub Street*," I say to myself for the one millionth time that day.

Day 1

As I embark on my diet, I decide to live as Jackie did and select white jeans and a turtleneck to wear, even though it is winter. In Jackie Kennedy's high school yearbook, she lists her favorite song as "Limehouse Blues" and her favorite saying as "Play the rhumba next." I listen to "Limehouse Blues" as I put on my jeans. It sounds like music that would play if you ever had a seizure in an amusement park. I like it!

I take a potato to work with me. Around 2:00 p.m., rather hungry, I microwave it within an inch of its life. It emerges shrunken and weirdly hard in some parts. I cut it open, slather it with sour cream and caviar, and take a bite. Despite the vagaries of the potato itself, it really is delicious. I would eat this at any sort of fancy occasion, including my birthday and my mother's birthday. I am not even hungry for many hours afterward, even though I do leave halfway through an 8:00 p.m. showing of *Anna Karenina*, possibly because I am too hungry to concentrate. But I also could have just hated it.

Day 2

I wake up really hungry. This is to be expected, but still I am surprised given how well the "one potato" thing was going yesterday. I put "Limehouse Blues" on, but it makes me feel jittery. I eat a potato at work, then pack up my caviar and assorted potato accessories and board a bus to Rhode Island, where I am spending Thanksgiving. I pack the caviar in ice and give it its own seat on the bus.

Day 3

I weigh myself in my childhood bathroom. I have lost three pounds in two days. This is a very effective diet! I am also crazy now, however. For example, I realize my tiny jar of caviar is basically empty. I gave an empty tin of caviar its own seat on the bus!

Day 4

Today is Thanksgiving. *Cooking for Madam* has a whole chapter about Thanksgiving, which Marta says was "opening day of the hunt" for the Kennedys. (Tallyho!) The menu is pretty traditional, so to honor Jackie specifically I choose a fruit dessert that Marta says Jackie preferred over other types of desserts. I make "Peaches Cardinal," which is basically steamed peaches and raspberry sauce. It is not as good as pie, and I am the only one who eats it. My mother promptly throws out the raspberry sauce, which has taken many hours to strain. "Play the rhumba next!" I almost say to her, but I don't.

Day 5

Today is my sister's birthday. We go to Newport, Rhode Island, the site of Jackie's wedding to JFK, and drive by the church they got married in. It is made out of brownstone and looks dark and imposing. I have mussels, another Jackie favorite, for lunch and try to imagine how to say "Play the rhumba next!" in a way that would not completely disrupt a conversation.

Day 6

After periods of heavy eating, Jackie would go on a fruit fast. Though my Thanksgiving binge also consisted of fruit, I do the fast anyway, which is not particularly terrible, dietwise. However, it is rather hard to eat fruit while everyone else is eating Thanksgiving leftovers. People rib you about diet journalism. Food is an emotional conundrum, after all. A paragraph in Marta's cookbook about Aristotle Onassis illustrates this maxim quite well. Apparently one day, Onassis arrived for dinner after everyone else had eaten. He asked Marta to pass the salt, and when she tried to hand it to him, he made her put it down on the table. Then he said, "If you hand someone salt, you will have a fight with them and I don't want to be fighting with you."

Day 7

Today I decide to make the dinner Jackie so lovingly supervised for when Lee Radziwill and her husband came to visit her in Washington. The menu involves *poulet à l'estragon* and casserole *marie blanche*. If you are not familiar with French (me), the casserole involves both sour cream and cottage cheese, and the chicken is basically made with oil and tarragon. At the time this was apparently the height of sophistication. At the party, everyone danced to an orchestra until 3:00 a.m. In her book *Grace and Power: The Private World of the Kennedy White House*, Sally Bedell Smith notes that the Kennedy-Radziwill party attendees sat at tables "covered in yellow linen with white, embroidered organdy top cloths, and decorated with low vermeil baskets of spring flowers." In my version of the party, my mom and I eat a disgusting casserole (I do not get combining sour cream with cottage cheese, yet this seems to be a bylaw of the 1960s) as we watch *Liz and Dick* on Lifetime.

Day 8

Back in New York, my poor friend and I make a dinner after Jackie's own heart: bay scallops with small strips of pepper and a spinach risotto. Jackie was a big fan of risotto, but I am concerned that this recipe does not incorporate cheese, which has been essential in most risottos I have loved. This is just rice mixed with spinach leaves I put in a blender. It is supposed to turn a "nice green color," and I guess it does, if that is a thing that food is supposed to do. It tastes like dirt. Marta said, "That was the thing about Madam and food. She was very refined about it in the ways she was about everything, but [dining] wasn't really what she was most interested in."

Days 9 and 10

I have just gotten to the part in Marta's cookbook where Jackie discovers Lean Cuisine. According to Marta, "she couldn't get over that you just had to put one in the oven and after a short time you took it out, and there was everything from soup to dessert. She thought that was great." I don't know what this means—soup and dessert, all in one Lean Cuisine? Are we eating the same Lean Cuisines? I buy a Lean Cuisine mac and cheese and microwave it for lunch. A suspicious amount of water collects at the bottom of the tray—soup?

Day 11

I am off the diet and feel both thinner and more refined. My white jeans even fit better, even though I will never wear them again. In the end, Jackie had impeccable taste, even in diet food. Despite the times in which she lived, she always ate pretty okay things and wrote such incredibly nice notes to Marta, including a particularly gushing one about mango sorbet. Diets, it turns out, can be elegant affairs. Play the rhumba next!

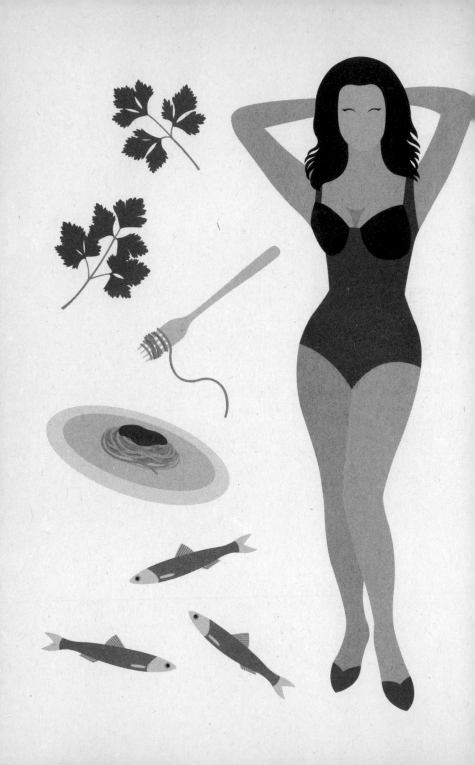

I Tried
Sophia Loren's Diet

According to legend, when asked what her beauty secrets were, famed Italian actress Sophia Loren was characteristically pithy: "Everything you see," she famously said, "I owe to spaghetti." In our current antigluten moment, such a sentiment might strike the modern ears as odd. "Pasta?" a modern woman might say while typing a code into her iPad. "Pasta can only lead to scurvy and an early grave. What of quinoa?"

Of course, in the modern era, Sophia denies actually saying that awesome thing about spaghetti. But it is true that Sophia has heavily extolled the magical healing powers of pasta. She wrote two pasta cookbooks. She wrote a book on beauty and mentioned pasta a lot. When people asked her, "Why did a twenty-eight-year-old Matt Damon hit on you at the Oscars?," she just smiled, but you knew she was thinking something about pasta. So the message was clear.

Sure, recently pasta has been demonized as fattening, sad, upsetting, and mean—but what if it's not? What if pasta is the greatest weight-loss food known to mankind? It would be impossible to know that without trying it, and this, dear readers, is what I will do for you. Because the public needs to know!

Preparation

There is actually quite a bit of information on what Sophia Loren ate. She produced two cookbooks herself and even wrote a self-help book called *Women & Beauty*, which is about beauty, nutrition, and fitness and is full of backhanded compliments about other actresses, like, "Take for instance Elizabeth Taylor or Barbra Streisand. The way they dress could not be described as conventionally elegant, yet they both have a unique sense of how they want to look."

I buy the self-help book, a book called *Sophia: Living and Loving: Her Own Story,* and the pasta cookbook entitled *Sophia Loren's Recipes & Memories.*

"Almost from the beginning, interviewers have asked me what diet I follow to stay in shape," said Loren in her cookbook. "It amuses me to see their expressions when I answer 'pasta.' It is only a slight exaggeration. I adore pasta and eat it almost every day." According to *Women & Beauty,* Loren really did eat a serving of pasta for lunch and dinner, followed occasionally with a lean meat or fish. I plan to do the same.

To be honest, I am kind of excited about this diet because it doesn't sound like a diet. Pasta for all meals? What could be better! Pasta is my favorite food, which I realize is not particularly original.

The problem is that recently, through no evidence at all, except for the Phantom of the Opera rash I had running down my face after I briefly cut out gluten on the Gwyneth diet, I have convinced myself I have a gluten allergy. Can I still eat pasta with my fake gluten allergy going on? It seems hard.

Day 1

Today is the day that I start the diet. I'm unusually excited, not just because I love pasta but also because I've always been a big fan of Sophia Loren. In high school I rented a movie that happened to be very influential on me called *What a Woman!* It starred Sophia Loren and Marcello Mastroianni and was dubbed in English. The whole movie is Sophia Loren getting mad at Marcello Mastroianni and then doing absolutely psycho things to show Marcello Mastroianni that she is mad. Then after that he yells, "What a woman!" and forgives her.

I start the diet off by making Loren's famous "Salsa Sophia," which I will spoon over whole wheat pasta per Loren's instructions (Loren says that whole wheat pasta is the healthiest pasta). It does seem to be a recipe that Sophia Loren actually made up (once you start reading her cookbook you realize a suspicious number of recipes actually originate with her cook). "Salsa Sophia" is similar to a pesto—a combination of anchovies, pine nuts, and a lot of parsley ground with a mortar and pestle. It's pretty delicious, and I have always especially liked anchovies. The catch comes when I actually look at the serving size of pasta Sophia is asking me to eat. It's about as small as a balled-up fist, which I have always heard is the actual serving size for pasta, even though I have never eaten such a portion. When I finish my helping of pasta I am starved, and in some ways hungrier than I have been when I forced myself to eat something disgusting, like tofu cheese or seed falafel. This diet might actually be harder than I thought.

Later, before going out to dinner and a show, I decide to peruse Sophia Loren's beauty tome *Women & Beauty* to get some tips.

To that end, I really scrub my head when I'm in the shower. ("Keep running the warm water through it until every last bit of soap is gone and the hair squeaks.") I put on a severe amount of eye makeup (eyes "deserve the most attention," says Sophia). Because it's a rather formal outing, I wear a dress I actually took to a tailor once. The problem is that because it fits correctly, it is not very comfortable. It's also electric blue, which Sophia would probably disapprove of. She, for example, thinks purple is too "violent" a color and used to dye all her clothing black, even her handkerchief.

For dinner before the show, I have a small helping of pasta and some shrimp and am again oddly starving. I don't really understand why. I'm sure this was enough food, technically, to survive. It's more that it was just so delicious, I actually want to keep eating it. I look longingly at the M&M's my companion eats during the show, but I control myself, as Sophia does not believe in the American habit of snacking. I also realize that whether I am actually allergic to gluten or whether I have made myself think I am allergic to gluten, I am fancying myself ill throughout the second act. Time to switch to gluten-free pasta?

Day 2

The next day, I continue to be hungry. I make myself an English muffin (Sophia likes them) and a scant hour and a half later decide to have my lunch, pasta in a lemon cream butter sauce. The pasta is very lemony and kind of bitter because you have to grate lemon rinds into the butter. Still, it's delicious. Too delicious to stop eating so prematurely! This is starting to remind me of when Sophia Loren's mother won a Greta Garbo look-alike contest and was promised a trip to America to have a screen test but then her mother (Sophia's grandmother) wouldn't let her go because she was worried that the Black Hand was going to murder her just like they murdered Rudolph

Valentino (even though Valentino died of appendicitis, but whatever). So Sophia Loren's mother had to stay in their tiny Italian town and eventually had an illegitimate child (Sophia) out of rebellion. An all-pasta diet seems great until it is ripped cruelly away from you.

In the afternoon, I decide to walk with my friend all around the city. Walking is Sophia's preferred mode of exercise, and she walks for a long time every day. At one point, my friend and I stop for a minute and both think about buying overalls. They are very in now. But then I remember how disappointed Sophia was when her niece wore clothing that Sophia found awful, like "baggy pants and strange tops that made her look like a farmer at Harvest time," and so I don't buy them.

For dinner, I try to make Sophia's tomato sauce over gluten-free pasta. I couldn't keep eating the whole wheat pasta. The rash never returned, but after reading a WebMD article about gluten intolerance I think I have all the symptoms on that page. I feel bad begging off Sophia's preferred pasta, but gluten-free pasta is far worse than regular pasta and this does seem to fit my estimation of Sophia's powers of self-denial. Cary Grant was always proposing to her and she always said no. One time her sister (who married Mussolini's son???) openly mused, "I sometimes wonder if Sophia today has any fun in her life."

As any Italian home cook knows, you are always ultimately judged on your tomato sauce. I decide to make Sophia's marinara tonight. Sophia's is pretty darn good, if a little less flavorful than what I am used to. It's very simple—just fresh tomatoes, herbs, and a little sugar. I myself am partial to gravylike sauces because I'm a philistine from Rhode Island.

Day 3

After a hearty (but small) breakfast of spaghetti carbonara, I decide to make a three-course Italian feast for dinner made entirely from the Sophia cookbook. I am going to make *pasta all'amatriciana* and veal saltimbocca. Unfortunately, the grocery store is out of veal, but as Sophia says, "Neapolitans live by instinct," so I decide on the fly to change my dish to chicken saltimbocca. Also, Anthony Quinn once aggressively kissed Sophia while she was eating a lamb chop, so I feel that she would appreciate the lack of red meat in the meal.

Luckily, the dinner is fantastic. The *pasta all'amatriciana* (which has bacon and pepper) is especially great. At the beginning of the meal, I decide to have the small helping of pasta the diet allows. But then the baby-fist-size portion just looks so sad and I remember when I went to a wine-tasting class in Italy and the instructor said, "There are no rules for wine!" and that was the whole class. "Oh screw it," I say, and help myself to a more American-size portion. I am off the diet. It's over!

So what did I learn? I learned that sometimes, the best things are terrible when they come in small packages. Better to live like a health nut and then the goodies of life aren't always right in front of your face. Sophia, for your moderation, I salute you! What a woman!

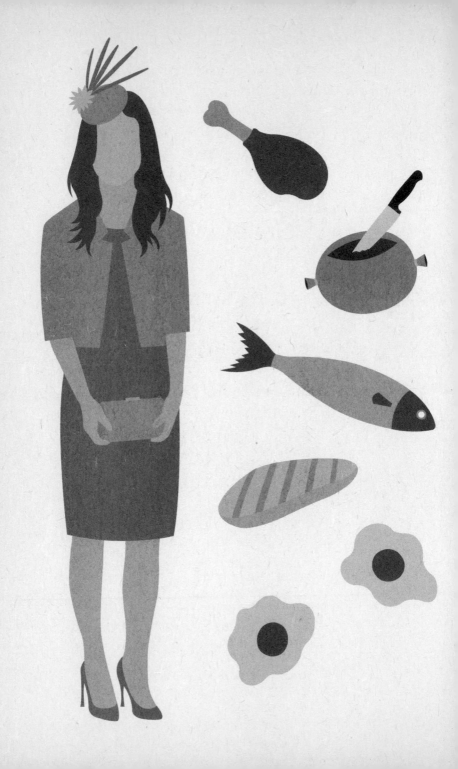

I Tried
Pippa Middleton's Diet

The public is very fickle in a stupid way, and Pippa Middleton is an excellent example of this. One minute you (Pippa Middleton) are wearing a beautiful dress at a wedding and everyone loves you and thinks you have a nice bum. Then, the next minute, you are in an extraordinarily small car with a group of handsome Frenchmen and one of them is holding a toy gun and suddenly you are the object of censure. What is a woman to do in such circumstances but write a reviled book about celebrating called *Celebrate* and then later pen an exercise column in the *Telegraph*? The public drove her to do it.

I, for one, have always been a fan of Pippa's lifestyle journalism and of the can-do spirit that allowed her to take her bum and turn it into a brand. I very much defended her when she was in that car with all those Frenchmen. They were all so handsome, and she had just gone to a historical ball with them.

Thus, it was with a particular pride that I decided to take up the diet and exercise regimens that fueled Pippa's rise to the top ranks of lifestyle journalism. If the *Daily Mail* is to be believed and the Middletons really are relentless social graspers and achieved their current position through hard work and patience, then I want them to teach me their dietetic secrets. Because I know nothing about any of those virtues, and I would like to marry a king.

Preparation

My diet will trace the life cycle of a Pippa Middleton, as that is truly the only way to understand how she has reacted to the slings and arrows of outrageous fortune. I will start my diet with the diet that Pippa followed right before her breakthrough appearance at the royal wedding: the Dukan Diet, a bestselling French program (the French—*always* the cause of one's rise and one's downfall!). I go ahead and buy the eponymous book at the bookstore. It looks both cheerful and scary at the same time. But I am not done! To complete my Pippa transformation, I buy her four-hundred-page book, *Celebrate*. This I will use to throw one of my famous dinner parties. I also discover all of Pippa's coverage of health fads for the *Telegraph*—a partner in arms! I will attempt every single one of these exercise fads, even though Pippa is definitely a better athlete than I am.

Day 1

The Dukan Diet is basically a French version of the Atkins Diet, an entirely protein affair with occasional breaks for dry and oil-less vegetables. Despite being a woman who loves diets and embraces them with two fists, I have never done any super-high-protein diets except for my brief dalliance with the diet of America's fattest president, William Howard Taft. And that was a disaster of epic proportions.

Dukan himself even seems ambivalent about bringing his fun French diet to the uncultured land of the free and the home of the brave. He starts his book off with a fun story about how he likes Americans because they saved the French from the Nazis, but eventually he confesses that Americans "scared [him] somewhat" because we are so fat. Luckily, he eventually realized that within "every North American citizen there is a human being who longs to respect the essential relationship between a healthy body and a healthy mind," and he decided to give us the diet after all.

I have decided to do the three "phases" of the diet in the next three days. Sure, this may be quick, but I feel it will give me the lay of the Dukan land. The first phase of the diet is the "attack phase." In the attack phase, you can eat only protein the entire day. This is actually completely fine because you don't have to do portion control; you can eat as much as you want. I have two eggs in the morning, a huge helping of sashimi for lunch (with only a splash of soy sauce), and several fillets of fish for dinner (I do cheat slightly and have a dumpling too). It feels great, honestly. No deprivation at all. Just a vague hatred of fish.

Day 2

Today I am in the "cruise" phase of the diet, a.k.a. the day when I can eat both unlimited amounts of protein and a series of unsatisfying vegetables. Really good vegetables such as potatoes are somehow never included, which is very annoying. For lunch, I am weirdly starving and have two grilled chicken breasts and some soppy mushrooms stewed in their own juices. At the end of this repast, I am full but bored.

For dinner, I decide to try one of the staples of the Dukan Diet—the infamous oat bran galette, which is a pancake or "galette" (French!) that is made out of bran, Greek yogurt, and an egg white. (I put some garlic in there, too. Mistake.) Dukan once served it to his daughter Maya and reports that she felt "completely full." Despite the fact that the pancake in its uncooked state looks a lot like yogurt with some garlic bits in it, the end result (after cooking it in an oil-less pan) is not that bad. It ends up looking like a regular pancake with some garlic bits in it. I top this with salmon and low-fat cream cheese. It reminds me of an extremely tasteless bagel.

Days 3 and 4

Today is a "consolidation day," i.e., a day in which I eat both protein and the occasional slice of whole wheat bread. I have my slice of bread in the morning with my egg. To be honest, I really do miss carbs, but not as much as I have missed food on other diets. I weigh myself and realize this particular undisciplined sort of eating does not work for me. I weigh the same. I celebrate this with the "celebration feast" Dukan allows in the cruise phase. At this dinner, I eat three different desserts because I am celebrating. I wonder, slightly, if this is what Dukan intended for me to do.

Day 5

Now done with the Dukan Diet, I decide to attempt Pippa's current career as a nutritional and lifestyle journalist (really, the best kind of journalist). Pippa used to write fairly frequently for the *Telegraph*. In each column, she did a crazy fad exercise regimen and then an unseen photographer took pictures of her in weird outfits. In one of her more recent columns, Pippa attempted a new French craze sweeping England called "hydrospinning," which is essentially a spin class in your own personal Jacuzzi. As Pippa puts it, "I like cycling. I really like Jacuzzis. But cycling in a Jacuzzi?" (This really is a good column, I have to tell you.) Unfortunately, we do not yet have the particularly French pastime of cycling in a Jacuzzi in New York City, but we do have the ability to do a spinning class in a communal pool with other people, which I eventually decide to do. We call it aqua cycling.

Unfortunately, I happen to show up at this aqua-cycling studio right at the nadir of the polar vortex. I am going to tell you something: I do not want to aqua-cycle during the polar vortex, even though I have to for science. I do not want to pay forty dollars to be submerged in a freezing pool. I have been wearing an outfit made entirely of fleece for several weeks. However, it isn't that horrible in practice. You can forget about arctic temperatures when you realize how hard it is to cycle in water. I could barely stay on the bike or move my legs. It reminded me of what it is like for me to ride a bike normally.

Days 6 and 7

After going up to New Haven to see my friend star in a production of *My Fair Lady* (Pippa would have done the same, I felt), I return to triumphantly hold a "Burns Night" for my friends. "What is Burns Night?" you ask? I found out about it when I read Pippa's book, *Celebrate*. A Burns Night is a night that celebrates Scotland. You are required to eat haggis at it, which, according to Pippa, is the "minced heart, lungs and liver of a sheep or calf mixed with beef fat, onions, oatmeal and seasonings." Delicious! Haggis happens to be illegal in New York City. Apparently you can't eat lung here. This is not the land of the free.

Before I even decide how to find illegal haggis (the streets?), I invite all my friends to a dinner party and send them a picture of haggis I found on Wikipedia. It looks like a huge piece of intestine with a hole in it. Everyone is excited about it, especially when I tell them I will order pizza if they come to the party. Eventually, I end up purchasing a legal version of haggis that does not have lung at a British grocery store.

Despite the fact that *Celebrate* is several hundred pages long, it is sometimes surprisingly vague. Pippa has no directions for the haggis other than heating it up in a pan and serving it with a turnip-and-potato mixture. I am wary of putting the haggis in a pan—it recently emerged from its tin in a series of congealed brown clumps—but it fries up rather nicely.

When my guests arrive, I give them a Scottish cocktail that involves oatmeal juice (oatmeal soaked in water and strained), honey, whiskey, and heavy cream. It is called Atholl Brose and is politely declined by all except me, because I sort of like it. It tastes like an old sweater, which is a comfort after all the aqua spinning. Luckily, however, the haggis is beloved. It tastes like a saltier version of corned beef hash. One of my especially ambitious friends even recites an ode to the haggis. I still order pizza like I promised, however.

Day 8

This morning, I decide to do a Zumba class at 9:00 a.m. It is a horrible existential experience. It reminds me of when, for Pippa's thirtieth birthday party, she decided to do a flamenco dance for everyone she had ever known. She described it thus: "I stomp my heels, I spin—I'm a little dizzy but before I know it, my hands have stretched to the sky, my head turns to one side and I pout dramatically as I hold my final position." I don't know about flamenco, but I cannot imagine doing public Zumba at my thirtieth birthday party.

Day 9

Still hopelessly following Pippa's *Telegraph* articles, I decide to take a boxing class. This is even worse than Zumba. I can't remember any of the boxing combinations, the instructor keeps yelling, "No!" at me, and all the men in the class are very handsome in the style of men in a car in France. They never forget any of the combinations.

After boxing, I decide to make Pippa's post-boxing meal, which combines spinach, pomegranate seeds, Peppadew peppers, feta cheese, allspice, and chicken. Weirdly, it is not all that bad. It's actually the best thing I have had on the diet and much better than the oat bran galette. It tastes like a very healthy version of sweet-and-sour chicken. I might make it for myself normally.

Day 10

For my last night of the Pippa diet, I wind up going to Catch, the restaurant she visited in New York when some people thought she was going to move here. It's so glamorous, like a club with food. There are so many lights!

Now that I'm finally off Pippa's punishing regimen, I must admit that I did enjoy it. Her recipes certainly weren't Gwyneth-level (what is?), but some really were surprisingly delicious. I never thought pomegranates would taste good with allspice, but they did. Also, I think a muscle is appearing in my leg.

In conclusion, Pippa could be riding around all the time with French people in motorcars but instead she is out there, trying to develop muscles in her legs. You've got to give the girl some credit.

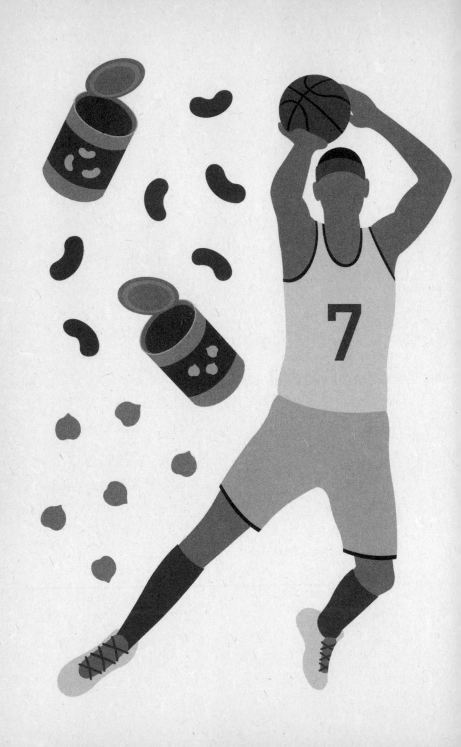

I Tried
Carmelo Anthony's Diet

Knicks player Carmelo Anthony once made headlines
when he told a group of sports reporters that he had
lately completed a fifteen-day spiritual cleanse called the
Daniel Fast and that it might have been affecting his play.

"I haven't had a good meal in about two and a half weeks.
No meats, no carbs, anything like that," Anthony told
reporters in an effort to explain why he had been averag-
ing only thirty-two points a game in January (this seems
pretty good to me, but what do I know?) and his shoot-
ing percentage was slightly down. Then a bunch of sports
journalists freaked out about it.

"I'm all for a good cleanse, but not in the middle of an NBA season," the New York *Daily News* opined. "Seriously, with the slow starts they've been having, I think it's a legitimate question as to whether Melo's fasting hurt the team," the *Wall Street Journal*'s Chris Herring tweeted. Knicks coach Mike Woodson eventually addressed the diet and ended up sounding like a Hollywood starlet's publicist, waving off anorexia concerns with diplomatic utterances about "the right foods" and having "faith" in Melo.

So how extreme is this diet? I would have to try the Daniel Fast and find out. Probably really extreme if all these newspapermen were making such a big deal out of it! They never exaggerate.

Preparation

The Daniel Fast is a diet based on passages in the biblical book of Daniel in which the eponymous prophet goes on several fasts. In one he eats only vegetables; in another he gives up "precious breads." The modern Daniel Fast allows whole grains but prohibits meat, dairy, coffee, alcohol, and sugar, i.e., all of the most delicious things in the world. Daniel Fasters describe their technique as "a vegan diet with even more restrictions." I decide to follow the fast's meal plan and recipes and play basketball for the next thirty-six hours to get a sense of what starving starlet Carmelo Anthony is going through.

Day 1

I start the day with a brisk shopping trip to buy ingredients for the recipes outlined on Daniel-Fast.com. The Daniel Fast advocates three square meals and two snacks a day (already this diet sounds pretty easy) but also maintains that "while we can eat as much food as we want and any time we want . . . we want to keep in mind that we are fasting." (Even easier.) I keep this in mind as I pay for my food.

When I get home I make the stir-fry, which is basically kale, onions, carrots, and soy sauce over rice. It's a little boring and does not have much protein but tastes decent. The portion is actually too big for me to eat all at once, so I eat half and save the rest.

Fortified by this important meal, I decide to go play basketball, which I have literally never done before in my life.

(I used to sit in the girls' bathroom during gym class. It was fun there!) I buy a basketball at Modell's and head to a court I find on the Internet. Carmelo says he needs only forty-five minutes in the gym each day to play as well as he does, so I plan to do the same. How hard can it be to shoot baskets for forty-five minutes a day? Very hard, it turns out, when you are really super bad at it. The ball keeps landing in a puddle of water vaguely near the court because that is the closest I can get it to the hoop. Repeatedly hurling a ball into the air and fetching it is so demoralizing (and wearying for my arms) that I download my first audiobook ever, *Safe Haven* by Nicholas Sparks, to distract myself.

For dinner, I have the rest of the stir-fry and some homemade flat bread called chapati that I make from flour and water. I am actually stuffed, despite eating about half the quantity of food I was supposed to eat. This diet is great!

Day 2

The most difficult part of the Daniel Fast is the lack of coffee. For breakfast, I have oatmeal and an atrocious headache. I distract myself by thinking about *Safe Haven*.

Why did Katie dye her hair brown even though she's a natural blonde? What is the dark secret haunting her? I need to know.

For lunch, I make a curry by combining one can of kidney beans, one can of garbanzo beans, one can of lentils, and several raisins. It's way too much food; I realize later that I made eight portions of this curry and I am only one woman. I eat about one-sixteenth of what I made and am stuffed. I'm going to be eating these leftovers forever.

At three thirty my caffeine-withdrawal headache is so bad that I break down and buy a tall black coffee at Starbucks. It is delicious and my headache immediately goes away, but I do experience guilt. However, it is imperative to not have a headache when playing a super-competitive game of basketball. This time, I invite two friends to the basketball court and we play Horse for forty-five minutes. I am the worst at it by far, but I have a lot of energy from all those beans.

I break my fast with a steak dinner, just as Carmelo Anthony did when he told a crowd of reporters, "I surrender." The steak is superlative, and I greatly enjoy the accompanying bread. I also surrender.

At the end of the Daniel Fast, I feel the usual relief one feels at the end of a diet. It is hard not to have a cookie when you want it. But does this diet deserve the consternation that many sports analysts gave it? Of this I am unsure.

Is the Daniel Fast boring? Yes. Does it get tiring to eat oodles of beans without much seasoning? Absolutely. Would this diet be even harder if you are a pro athlete of Carmelo Anthony's stature and skill level? With my new appreciation for the difficulty of throwing a large orange ball through a circular net atop a pole, I suspect so. But is this worse than what Jackie and Marilyn had to put up with their whole lives? Does it hold a candle to the travails of dietetic folk hero Gwyneth Paltrow? Absolutely not! In conclusion, men are babies when it comes to diets. NBA superstars are less hard-core than the average American teen girl the week before prom!

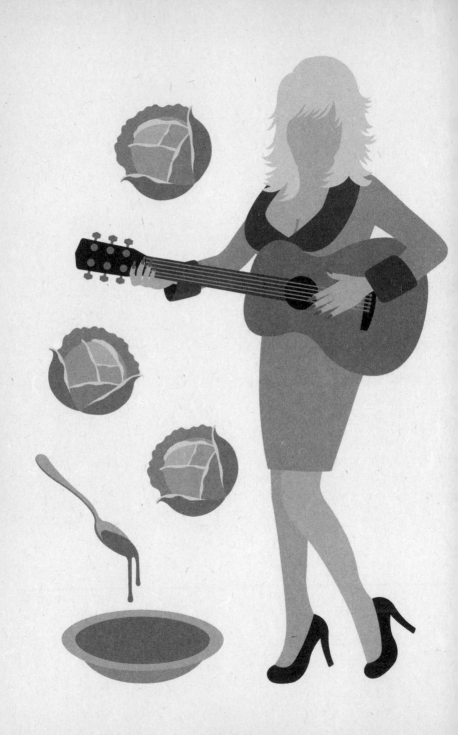

I Tried
Dolly Parton's Diet

I tried every diet in the book," Dolly Parton, a woman after my own heart, once said. "I tried some that weren't in the book. I tried eating the book. It tasted better than most of the diets."

But Dolly does have a subtle and interesting distinction in the world of dieting. She actually has an iconic diet named after her. The Cabbage Soup Diet is also known as the Dolly Parton Diet and sometimes known as the TWA Stewardess Diet (?). I didn't know that either until I googled "Dolly Parton" and "Diet" together. The more you know.

I have never actually seen any evidence that Dolly did the Cabbage Soup Diet in particular. She did say that she once saw a diet named after her in a magazine and tried it. "It had nothing to do with me," she told *People* magazine. "But I thought I might as well see if I can lose weight on my own diet." And hopefully the Cabbage Soup Diet was what she was referring to? I don't know.

Preparation

The Cabbage Soup Diet looks incredibly, incredibly gross. If you look up pictures of cabbage soup online you will see what I mean. It looks like a poisonous stew that would kill someone in the last act of a medieval play, and it is an odd magenta color because of the canned tomatoes in it.

Apparently, you usually have to go on the Cabbage Soup Diet for seven days, but I decide to do it for only two. Cabbage soup allegedly is quite violent to your digestive system. I'm sure Dolly would agree that brevity is probably best in these circumstances.

It's not like you are only eating cabbage soup on the Cabbage Soup / Dolly Parton / TWA Stewardess Diet. You can eat other things! One of the days, you can have some fruit along with your cabbage soup. Another day you can have some vegetables and as much cabbage soup as a girl could possibly want! You can also have a baked potato on the vegetable day, but Dolly once said that every time she ever "fell off of" a diet, it was because of potatoes. So I will probably avoid them.

Day 1

The general order of the Cabbage Soup Diet is 1) cabbage soup with only fruit, 2) cabbage soup with only vegetables. You are supposed to do the fruit day first, but I switch it up because vegetables work better for me the first day. I have to go out to lunch and dinner, and ordering vegetables is far less obnoxious than asking for a fruit plate. Ordering a fruit plate is just asking people to hate you (veteran dieters, take note!).

In the morning, I decide to make my first batch of cabbage soup. I chop up an entire head of cabbage and combine it with canned tomatoes, onions, carrots, and a slight pinch of garlic. While it is cooking, I open a window. It smells like burnt rubber, which is not something you would necessarily associate with cabbage.

After that, I decide to go out to lunch. When Dolly goes out to lunch, sometimes men spontaneously erupt in applause and Dolly says things like, "I don't even know them." When I go to lunch, I realize that I forgot I left cabbage soup on the stovetop with the stove still on. It dawns on me when I am about an hour into a non-applause-ridden repast of unadorned carrot. I excuse myself to my lunch friend and rush home to the pot and realize that, though reduced, the soup still exists and did not burn down the apartment. I am relieved, and as a treat I serve myself a bowl of cabbage soup. It tastes like boiled cabbage with ketchup on it.

Later that evening, over a plate of boiled okra and cauliflower (Dolly likes okra but only the fried kind), I think about Dolly and her mysterious husband, Carl. No member of the public has seen Carl for forty years. Apparently Carl has only seen Dolly perform once. His likeness is not even in Dollywood (the Dolly Parton theme park). Dolly put it this way: "Carl said, 'I want to go up there any time I want, and I don't want somebody coming out of the museum and telling me, 'You're Carl.'"

Dolly tells many stories about Carl, despite his ostensible absence. When she is at home with him she "teases her hair and puts it up in a little scrunchie." I try to do the same thing for my boyfriend, but he does not seem to notice or care about it.

Day 2

In the morning (I don't wake up at 2:30 a.m. like Dolly does; I wake up at a decent hour), the cabbage soup has settled into a congealed mess. I have to open three windows in my apartment just to air out the scent of the soup, and even then you can still smell it in the hall outside my apartment. I feel bad for my neighbors. I make the executive decision that I cannot handle the soup for breakfast.

When I finally arrive at brunch, I confine myself to a huge bowl of fruit, like some kind of saint. At around 2:00 p.m. I force myself to have a smidgen of cabbage soup. The cabbage has disintegrated into the soup and has become one with the broth. How is this possible? It seemed so solid yesterday. It is as shocking as the fact that Dolly is Miley Cyrus's godmother!

At least I can take refuge in living like Dolly. She once famously said, "It takes a lot of money to look this cheap," and with that in mind, I start wearing a small minidress I once bought from American Apparel around the apartment. I have always been too embarrassed to wear that dress in the light of day. I pair it with towering shoes and look at the cabbage soup bubbling in its pot, even though there is no heat source interacting with it. While wearing the minidress, I can see why Dolly is so militant about diets and plastic surgery. These spandex tubes are unforgiving. At one point she said, "If I have one more face-lift I'll have a beard!"

After eating some fruit (and some vegetables too, breaking the rules slightly) I decide to swallow some more cabbage soup. It is the only food I have in the house except some seeds left over from the Posh diet. But as I reheat the cabbage soup, I realize that I can't take it anymore. I have taken on too much! I will always love you, cabbage soup, but I will mostly hate you. I try to pour it into a plastic bag, but only some of it lands in the plastic bag and most of it lands on the kitchen floor. Now my kitchen smells of cabbage.

Day 3

Several days later (Dolly likes to take weekends off her diet but I took a few days more than that because I was cleaning the cabbage soup off of my floor), I decide to attempt a dieting tip Dolly advertised in her autobiography: chewing her food but not actually swallowing it. As Dolly says, "The pleasure and satisfaction is in the tasting and chewing." Is it? I don't know. I make my first attempt with a mound of tortilla chips. I put them in my mouth, chew them, and spit them out. It does not feel particularly pleasurable or satisfying. It is like chewing tortilla-chip-flavored gum. Gross food makes you not want to eat, but spitting out food seems like a crime! I end up eating the whole mound of tortilla chips.

I lost a bunch of weight on the Cabbage Soup Diet, but I also lost something more important—the ability to be in my kitchen for any length of time without smelling like cabbage. Dolly may have been a trailblazer in music, plastic surgery, and even the theme park business, but her diets make me want to escape to Dollywood and never return.

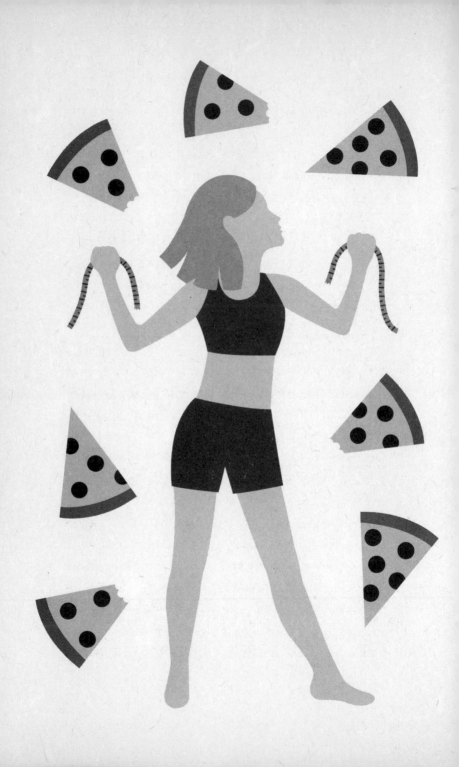

And Now,
a Slice of Pizza

Well, it is finally over. The dieting and depravity of the famous has at last been done, and I can't say I'm particularly disappointed. It was hard being on a diet at all times. I'm actually eating a piece of pizza as I write this, and it is a great relief to me.

But I started this journey of dieting with some specific questions in mind. Namely: Was I going to have any friends left at the end of the diet-athon? (No, the quail broke them.) Was I going to permanently change my body? (No! I weigh exactly the same as I did when I first started dieting. I don't know why this is. Every time I would diet I usually lost weight, but I almost immediately gained the weight back after eating one slice of pizza. I am probably gaining weight right now.) Which celebrity would I like the best? (A three-way tie between

Liz Taylor, Karl Lagerfeld, and the inimitable Gwyneth.
Liz because she was so glamorous, Karl because we both
think childhood was a time of endless stupidity, and
Gwyneth because she is the best at dieting and that's
very fun.) Which celebrity would I like the least? (Greta
Garbo, because what? She is crazy.) And what did I learn
about dieting? (I don't really know. Put eggs where they
don't need to be. Make seeds into falafel. Just do it!)

I think the main thing I realized is how terribly hard
it is to be an "ideal" woman at any time in history. I can't
even believe how many articles I have read in my life where
someone argues that the Golden Age of Hollywood had
more realistic body standards for women. And although
technically our ideal woman has gotten skinnier, there
was no time that was particularly great for women and
dieting. Even classic movie stars ate like insane people. In
fact, no time in Western history is necessarily safe from
diets since the Greeks basically made them up.

Really, instead of derision, these celebrities need
compassion! Their lives are horrible! They can literally
lose all their friends in one day because they made quail
and then they have to fight to get them back. And there
is intolerable pressure for them to look a certain way and
there is intolerable pressure for us to look like them. It
really is a cold war. But it really shouldn't be! What we
should all know is that every woman's life is hard and we
should be united in our trudge toward second-class citi-

zenship and hunger forever. I mean, sure, some men diet too, but it's just to wear the slim suits of Hedi Slimane. And they get paid better! That's really not the same thing.

Honestly, I was surprised at how much insight I gained about my favorite famous people when writing about them. I never quite imagined I would understand so much about the women I profiled through their food. Jackie Kennedy was very refined. Liz Taylor just wanted to drink! Gwyneth is great at everything, even healthy eating. Posh Spice has an almost devilish sense of humor. Cameron Diaz seems very sincere. I had a certain affinity for all of them after a while.

So, are you what you eat? Well, it's hard to say. I think you can gain tremendous understanding and almost an odd compassion for someone when you eat like them. You learn their vulnerabilities and little oddities and obsessions. You fully enter their world and you don't judge it. So, no but yes, as with most things.

Acknowledgments

First and foremost, I have to thank my editors at *New York* magazine. Maureen O'Connor, Kurt Soller, and Molly Fischer were completely invaluable to this project. These columns wouldn't be anywhere without their encouragement, hard work, and creativity. Thank you all for being such fantastic, patient, encouraging people. I should also acknowlege the excellent and talented Stella Bugbee for her endless kindness and support.

This book would not even exist without my editor at Vintage, Jenny Jackson. I would be nowhere without her general brilliance and tireless work ethic. Her vision for this project was so clear and intelligent, and she worked with me at all hours of the day and night to get it finished. She was integral to the tone, shape, and vision for this book. Plus, she's just hilarious and awesome! Thank you!

I also have to thank the team at Lutyens of Rubinstein, especially Jane Finigan for being a fantastic agent, and David Forrer at Inkwell, who did a great job putting this all together.

Finally, I need to thank my family—my mother, the first person I ever bounce anything off (for her invariably correct opinion), and my grandfather, who is basically the brains behind this entire operation. Thank you to William and Allison for their tremendous promotional skills and to my father for his courage in bookstores of all stripes. My friends, of course, need no introduction. I keep torturing them with horrid food and they keep coming back for more. They are the real heroes.